THE UNION EPIDEMIC

A Prescription for Supervisors

Warren H. Chaney, Ph. D.

and

Thomas R. Beech, J. D.

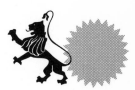

ASPEN SYSTEMS CORPORATION
GERMANTOWN, MARYLAND
1976

"This publication is designed to provide accurate and authoritative information in regard to the Subject Matter covered. It is sold with the understanding that the publisher is not engaged in rendering legal, accounting, or other professional service. If legal advice or other expert assistance is required, the services of a competent professional person should be sought." From a Declaration of Principles jointly adopted by a Committee of the American Bar Association and a Committee of Publishers and Associations.

Library of Congress Catalog Card Number: 76-24132
ISBN:0-912862-28-9

Printed in the United States of America

1 2 3 4 5

DEDICATION

A secret ballot election at any health care facility, conducted by the National Labor Relations Board, is a bitter contest. The only way management can win a struggle against professional union organizers is to put forth a real team effort on behalf of administration, department heads and every front-line supervisor. Therefore, this book is dedicated to those who work to win the battle to keep health care facilities for patients and not for the glory of union power and strife.

TABLE OF CONTENTS

PREFACE

There is no greater threat facing the health care industry today than the spread of the union epidemic. According to the National Labor Relations Board, unions won only forty-eight percent of the total board-conducted elections in 1975. This, the board reports, is the lowest percentage of union victories in the board's forty-year history. The health care industry, however, did not fare so well. Between August 1974, and the end of April 1975, the union success in health care industry elections was sixty-two percent. Strikes, slowdowns, and other work stoppages threatened the very core of health care in such states as New York, Hawaii, California, and Texas. Sadly, the patients suffered the most. They bore the brunt of "refusal of care" and a dramatic rise in costs, a direct result of unionization.

It is painfully obvious that the primary intention of unions is to organize the nation's health care employees, professional and nonprofessional alike. The sheer number of such people represent unimaginable sums of union membership dues and fees, and the unions have crawled out of the woodwork as starving mice after the cheese. The AFL-CIO, the Teamsters, and even professional associations such as the American Nurses Association are all scrambling for their share of the money pie.

In the authors' experience, no set of managers and supervisors within our country is less qualified to fight the union war and win than are those in health care: the experience of health care management does not stack well against the warriors on the union side. As a result, health care management gets caught up in the fear and confusion of an election. And not knowing when to call for help, they lose the battle.

The authors have found that management failure is the primary cause of union election success. Organizations deserve the unions they get. We realize this sounds hard, but it is true. Consequently, this book has been divided into two major sections. Section I deals with the union war once it has begun in your facility. It contains the necessary information and advice to recognize and resist the initial union organizational attempt. Its purpose is to assist you to wage the war against the union adversary successfully. It is recommended that this section be read before proceeding to section II.

Section II is concerned with taking the steps necessary to prevent unionism: "an ounce of prevention is worth a pound of cure." The primary cause of unionism is discussed, and prescriptions for cure are provided.

The authors sincerely hope *The Union Epidemic* will serve as a basic tool to halt and perhaps even retard the spread of unionism in an industry which we believe already suffers from overregulation. It is the authors' firm belief that unionization of health care is not inevitable. As a cancer, it can be curtailed. As the plague, it can be stopped.

Warren H. Chaney
Thomas R. Beech
Houston, Texas
October 1976

Section I
FIGHTING THE UNION BATTLE

Chapter 1

FRONT DOOR'S OPEN, GOOD BUDDY
or
UNION'S A-COMIN'

It is interesting to note that the basic causes of the labor revolts of over a century ago in the great union movements are still with us today. It is easy for health care administrators and supervisors to label the unions as troublemakers, agitators, outside power-mongers, and liars, but another thing for supervisors to see their own faults as reasons for the current successes by labor unions to organize health care employees.

Without doubt the primary reason for unionization in health care facilities is management failure. This might be hard to swallow, but it is true. This failure is usually a result of a number of subfactors such as economic problems, work problems, communication problems, and so on. But in every case of successful unionization it has been management that has failed to understand and responsibly fulfill its employees' needs and wants.

Incredibly enough, management has overlooked the *one* way to prevent unionism: to give employees those things that are ordinarily promised by unions. Instead, administrators seek to avoid unionism by various legal tactics, still maintaining the status quo. In the authors' experience this only forestalls the inevitable. Such management strategy is shortsighted. Even if successful in the first election, the union will certainly win the second time around. It is interesting to note that many of the unions refer to themselves as "second time winners."

You have your own personal feelings about labor unions. You probably have relatives and friends in a labor union. Depending on their personal experiences, that of others you have heard about or read about in the newspapers, and many other bits of information, you have formed a personal opinion. You are certainly entitled to it. However, this book is intended to provide you, as a supervisor, with necessary information about this new element in your working life. Since you are a supervisor you are a part of management's team in any union organizational attempt.

The law rightly recognizes that supervisors are an employer's best weapon to resist the union attempt to organize more dues-paying members. In all fairness, regardless of your own views on unions, a main function and purpose of every labor union in the United States is to organize new workers into full-fledged union members. A union depends on numbers for both power and finances. Readers must recognize that power motivates men as much as money, and in a hospital's campaign against unionization this theme must be utilized.

We have often been asked, "Don't some employees need a union?" Our answer is loud and clear—"no." But some employers deserve a union; i.e., if an employer and the supervisors do not care enough to try to understand, communicate with, and properly supervise others, then the union should win the election.

All the union needs to do is to get thirty percent of employees in a unit to sign union authorization cards. The union is then entitled to a government controlled and supervised secret ballot election. The organizer sees such elections as the report card of success for his/her employer—the union. The organizer is also allowed by law to deal directly with your employees; in their homes, a union meeting hall, a restaurant, or even a bar. The employer-hospital is not allowed to enlist any employees to campaign for its position (that a union is not needed), but it can use its supervisors, talking to employees to state management's position.

The hospital legally can require supervisors to assist it to remain nonunion. In all practicality, it must use such help to stand any chance at the National Labor Relations Board (NLRB) vote taken on election day. By the time the hospital learns that professional union organizers are seriously interested in organizing its employees, the union team, in almost every case, is already way ahead in successfully convincing employees that they need union representation.

Upon first hearing of union activity, the hospital should take a series of corrective and preventative actions. All supervisors must get involved in this process as early as possible. If you, as a supervisor, cannot do this because of personal views or any other reason, it is time to resign and return to employee status. If you do not, and try to "fake" it by giving lip service to the hospital's position, the hospital usually finds out; then you deserve to be fired. So start out honestly and make a commitment to do your job as a supervisor by explaining and presenting the hospital's position on the union to your employees.

The National Labor Relations Act specifically provides for and protects the right of management to resist unionization by actively campaigning among its employees. The union has a similar right to present its campaign materials. Campaign is a choice word for the battle to come, because the only objective is to convince enough voters for your side to win—to win the minds of people. It is a war of propaganda and counterpropaganda used by both hospital and union. It is much like a hot and bitter political election.

Rightfully you may ask what is all this fuss about, and what is in it for me? Well, as a supervisor, you had better be prepared for trouble. During the union's organizational drive, nasty rumors will be started by prounion employees; rumors that will involve supervisors; rumors that can deal with sexual affairs or other personal matters.

Your employees will be divided into two camps, the prounion employees might gather in small groups and stop talking whenever you pass by. Work-related complaints will increase among the union employees, and many will neglect work to engage in conversations with other employees in an effort to enlist them into the union camp.

During the union's organizational drive, you will have to maintain control and discipline. Much has been written and much has been said about the need for proper documentation. In fact, too much has been said recently about documentation. It is no longer true that supervisors are uninformed about the importance of proper documentation; now the problem is overdocumentation.

No one bothers to explain the fundamental objectives and goals to which documentation relates. When something happens, therefore, a supervisor typically believes it best to write down every minute detail or every possible reason to justify his/her action. For example, in the discharge of a two-year housekeeping

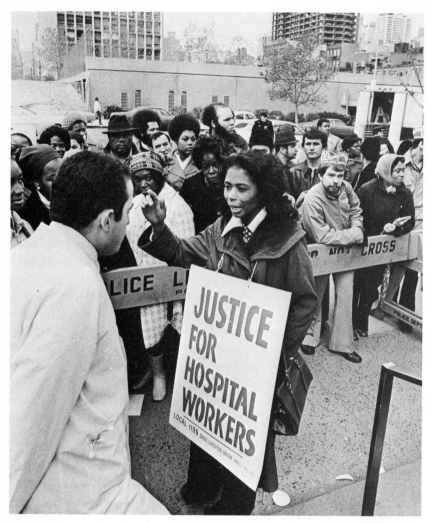

Tyrone Dukes/NYT Pictures

A picket arguing with a physician near the entrance to N.Y.U. Medical Center.

employee, the supervisor documented the following four reasons
for termination:

1. insurbordination,
2. refusing to follow instructions,
3. absenteeism, and
4. bad work performance.

The supervisor had instructed the employee to wash windows, at which time the employee refused and stated it was not her job. The employee was black; and when warned of discharge threatened to file a charge with the Equal Employment Opportunity Commission (EEOC). The supervisor got nervous, went to the personnel director, and they both reviewed the employee's personnel file and all records. Since the employee had several written warnings of excessive absenteeism, they decided to bolster the discharge by referring to it as one of the reasons for termination. For the same reason, bad work performance was also listed.

The problem arose when an EEOC investigation revealed that some presently employed white employees had more warnings of absenteeism or more warnings of bad work performance than the black employee, and no action of any kind was taken. Worse yet, it found that a white housekeeper also had refused previously to wash windows and that she was merely given a written warning.

Past practice plays an important role under all the various federal and state laws regarding employment practices. It makes sense to try and find out what an employer did under a similar factual situation in the past. If another employee was treated differently, it is natural to ask why. The hospital's answer is not improved by writing up weak or tenuous reasons for the particular action under review or investigation.

In a typical discharge situation, the best advice is to base the termination on one good ground, or possibly two grounds, but rarely any more than that. In other words: document the most important reason for the discharge, and keep it simple. Otherwise, when the discharge is investigated, a weakness in any one of the stated reasons for the termination creates a suspicion and casts doubts on the other reasons stated, even though the remaining reasons are all perfectly valid and well documented.

Whenever possible, take any serious job action with the employee in the presence of at least one other credible witness. If you do not, do not be surprised should you hear the former employee swear in court to a completely different version of what you said. A witness will not guarantee that the employee's version will still not be accepted, especially when dealing with federal agencies with a built-in bias such as the NLRB or the EEOC. But still, the witness certainly will strengthen your case.

In NLRB hearings, the hospital administrator will be present when the employee testifies to what you said and did. Even your firmest denial might not remove some doubts in the administrator's mind as to who is really telling the truth from the witness stand. With a witness supporting your facts, however, your superiors will feel better about it.

In addition, always keep your discharge conference with the employee brief and to the point. Certainly it is difficult for most of us to terminate any employee, especially a long term employee. In most cases it should not take more than ten to twenty minutes to complete the discharge procedure. Any longer time usually results in rehashing your grounds for the discharge, more denials from the employee, and, too often, angry words and arguments. Just say you're sorry, but the termination is final and effective immediately or with notice (if notice is required by your personnel policies). But end the conversation.

As a supervisor you must know and understand your hospital personnel policies on discipline and discharge. If such policies require a step process before termination, such as a written warning or a three-day suspension before discharge, follow it. Any deviation from such policy will provide ammunition for some government investigator that your action was unwarranted.

Government investigators normally look closely at due process, or their personal sense of common fairness to the employee. In other words, was the employee warned by written policy or hospital practice that such conduct would result in discipline or discharge? It is basic that an employee should be provided with actual knowledge of the prohibited conduct before being discharged for a violation of that conduct. So look at your disciplinary actions closely, and try to be fair before taking any drastic action.

Chapter 2

THE EPIDEMIC
or
THE SPREAD OF THE UNION DISEASE

To fight a war successfully a general must first understand why there is a war. To fight a union successfully, the health care supervisor must understand why the union is at his/her front door, and something of the history of that union. The purpose of this chapter is to provide some of that background.

The health care industry has been a recent target for unionization because it is one of the fastest growing industries in the nation. Today, unionization of health care professionals and non-professionals is no longer a simple threat; it is a complex reality with which administrators and supervisors must learn to cope. Collective employee activity in the health services sector of the nation's economy approximately doubled from 1961 through 1967. In the subsequent three years, this number doubled once again.[1] By the end of 1975 over twenty percent of all hospital employees were represented by some type of labor organization. This chapter will first examine the legislation behind the recent explosion in hospital labor organizations.

LEGISLATION RESULTING IN LABOR UNIONS

To appreciate the recent amendments of the federal labor laws concerning health care institutions, it is best to look at the first federal labor law passed in 1935, more commonly referred to as the Wagner Act. This legislation created many new procedures in the field of labor relations. Primarily, the law

1. delineates those employees and organizations considered to be under the act;

2. specifies the duties of the National Labor Relations Board (NLRB), charged with the administration of the act;
3. describes the rights of employees;
4. delineates management's unfair labor practices;
5. specifies procedures for selecting representatives, designating bargaining units, and conducting elections;
6. empowers the NLRB with authority to determine what are unfair labor practices and provide methods to seek redress and conduct investigations;
7. creates the Federal Mediation and Conciliation Service (FMCS) and specifies its duties;
8. denotes procedures that should be taken in national emergency disputes; and
9. describes how and under what conditions suits can be brought by and against labor unions and employers.[2]

Originally, the Wagner Act did not specifically exempt charitable, religious, or educational institutions from its jurisdiction. The particular status of voluntary nonprofit hospitals under the act was first considered when two unions filed a petition to represent the employees of Central Dispensary and Emergency Hospital in Washington, D.C.[3] The hospital appealed to be excluded from the NLRA because

1. hospitals were not engaged in trade, traffic, or commerce as defined in the legislation;
2. hospitals were nonprofit, and the law designated only profit-making enterprises; and
3. hospital activities were semipublic in nature and should be treated as an extension of the government.[4]

In a hearing soon after this appeal was made the NLRB denied the hospital's petition and ruled that voluntary nonprofit hospitals were within the jurisdiction of the Wagner Act. The NLRB stated that the hospital was engaged in interstate commerce and that the specific intent of the act was not based upon a profit motive. An appeal was filed, and the answer from a federal court stated:

"the hospital argues that the spirit or policy of the Act is such that we should read into it an exemption of charitable hospitals . . . . We cannot understand what considerations of public policy deprive hospital employees of the privilege granted to the employees of other institutions. The opinions, . . . holding that charitable hospitals and their nonprofessional employees are subject to the labor relations acts of those states, present what seems to us the only tenable view. . . ."[5]

This final statement appeared to have solved the status of hospital employees.

With the passing of the Wagner Act in 1935, the United States saw labor organizations grow by leaps and bounds. In 1935, there were 3.6 million members of labor unions. By 1947, members numbered 14 million. This boom was attributed to several factors, including the improving economic climate, the liberal sentiments of the times, dynamic union leadership, and most assuredly the NLRB. By the mid-1940s, as unions grew more prestigious due to their increasing size, people began to turn against unionism. The organizations, calling strikes at any provocation, made the general public feel that the Wagner Act had been too one-sided in favor of labor.[6]

Labor-Management Relations Act of 1947

In an effort to quell the complaints of the public, Congress, despite the fact it had to override a veto by President Harry S. Truman, passed the Labor-Management Relations Act (Taft-Hartley Act) of 1947. Among the important changes made by the Taft-Hartley Act was the inclusion of union unfair labor practices. In addition, the Wagner Act was amended so as not to include within its jurisdiction, " . . .the United States as any wholly owned government corporation, . . . or any state or political subdivision thereof, or any corporation or association operating a hospital if no part of the net earnings insures to the benefit of any private shareholder or individual. . . ."[7]

The Taft-Hartley Act made it clear that nonprofit hospitals had no legal obligation to recognize or bargain with their

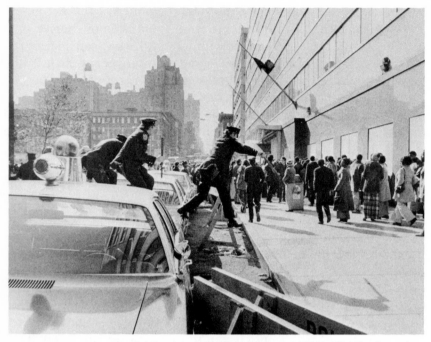

New York Post photograph by Richard Gummere © 1973, New York Post Corporation.

Cops jump over radio car to intercept striking hospital workers who had been throwing bottles at truck making oil delivery to Mount Sinai Hospital.

employees. In addition, hospital management was allowed to discharge union organizers or employees sympathetic to the unions.

Executive Order 10988-1961 and 11491-1969

During the past two and a half decades health care industry labor and management relations have changed considerably. Employee-employer interaction and legislative control have increased. Employees of federal hospitals are now subject to the provisions of Executive Order 10988, proposed by President John F. Kennedy in 1960. This order, enacted in June of 1961, recognized the rights of employees to seek collective recognition and bargaining rights with federal agencies and departments. The order also established the mechanisms through which employees should seek recognition and provisions under which unfair labor practices would be noted. In October of 1969, President Richard M. Nixon issued Executive Order 11491, which superseded the previous order and brought federal employee relations more in line with the provisions of the Taft-Hartley Act. Federal employees were still denied the right to strike.

State and local hospitals, prior to recent amendments of the federal labor laws, came under the protection of public employee bargaining units set up to represent the public employees of a particular state. In 1969, approximately thirty-seven states offered such protection for its public employees.[8] Nursing homes and proprietary hospitals have been subject to various court interpretations of the law; but nonprofit hospitals, although excluded from the provisions of the federal labor laws, were often subject to the jurisdiction of conflicting state labor laws.[9]

Public Law 93-360

Despite many attempts to define the rights and privileges of hospital employees, several labor unions lobbied in Washington for the same recognition granted to employees in private industry. Thus on July 26, 1974, Public Law 93-360 was enacted. It amended the federal labor laws to extend guaranteed uniform coverage to all nonpublic health care facilities. Simply put, it states that employees of health care facilities (except federal facilities) have every right to organize, collectively gather, and petition for more benefits, higher pay, or better working conditions. For the first time, all nongovernmental hospitals, nursing homes, clinics, health maintenance organizations, homes for the aged, and other institutions devoted to the care of infirm or aged persons are brought under the nation's labor laws.[10]

BARGAINING UNITS IN HEALTH CARE

Once collective bargaining in health care became a reality, both labor and management soon understood the need for precise understanding of the rules and regulations they had to follow. The National Labor Relations Act grants protection to health care employees to organize into appropriate bargaining units and to hold elections so the selection of a particular union can be made. This selection is of critical importance since it establishes the boundaries of the labor-management relationship.

The National Labor Relations Board is authorized to define the units appropriate for bargaining to insure employees all the freedoms granted by its sponsoring act. On May 5, 1975, the NLRB handed down a series of decisions that clarified and defined appropriate bargaining units in the health care field. The board ruled that the health care industry must deal with the following five units: (1) registered nurses; (2) all other professionals; (3) service and maintenance employees; (4) business office clerical employees; and (5) technical employees, including licensed practical nurses.[11]

Although these specific bargaining units have been established by the NLRB, there remain several specific restrictions. First, supervisors are not considered as employees under the coverage of the act. The definition of supervisor is indeed important because it is the supervisor who is the link between management and employees. In effect, supervisors are directly responsible for the application of the labor laws to his/her department.

A new section added to the National Labor Relations Act (NLRA) pertains directly to health care facilities. It states that a labor organization is prohibited from striking without giving ten days notice of the intention to strike management. This advance notice is to provide management with an opportunity to make arrangements for continued patient care, even if on a limited basis. Unions and health care facilities are also required by law to notify each other no less than ninety days before a contract modification or termination. The Federal Mediation and Conciliation Service (FMCS), which is the official mediator of a disagreement, must be given no less than sixty days notice of contract modification or termination. Before the 1974 amendments disputing parties were not forced to engage in mediation. However, due to the inclusion of specific provisions for health care facilities under the Taft-Hartley Act, labor and health care management are required to engage in mediation.[12]

Although other provisions are made in the amendments concerning health care facilities, the ones mentioned will provide a basic understanding for the remaining portions of this book.

Despite the fact that this chapter does not study all the legal aspects of the NLRA and its recent amendments, it is clear that health care administrators will be forced to become totally familiar with all legal ramifications. Labor unions have experience in organizing, strikes, contract negotiations, and grievances; health care management will be playing a whole new game, a game in which any error could have a drastic effect on labor relations.

Since the passing of Public Law 93-360, the medical literature has been flooded with articles concerning the expected surge in unions. Since employees now have the "green light" to organize, the twenty percent figure of employees represented by unions is expected to increase dramatically. However, before hospital employees begin to unionize in great numbers, one critical issue must be answered: should hospital employees, by virtue of the fact that they are members of a skilled profession, unionize? The implications of professionals joining unions in mass is being studied carefully not only by management but also by the professional organizations themselves.

UNIONIZATION OF PROFESSIONALS

Now that the application of the federal labor law to hospitals has been clarified by Public Law 93-360, the next question to be addressed by hospital employees is the ethical and moral ramifications involved in unionizing.

The professional and white collar employees have long viewed themselves as being above unionization. Labor unions were felt to be for factory and production workers, not for educated professionals. Professional workers could fend for themselves; but the factory worker, because of his limited educational background, had less bargaining power. Formerly, a professional's union membership could impede personal progress and career growth. But rapid technological and social changes are forcing this idea into obsolescence. Many well-informed people now believe that the United States is about to witness a surge of unionization among professionals.

Many feel, however, that health care professionals have no need for unions because, unlike others, they chose their profession

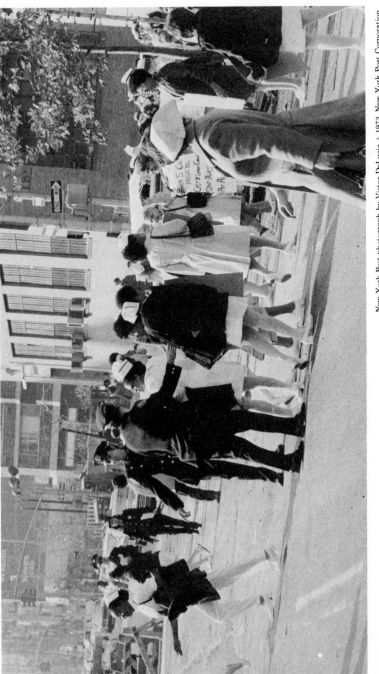

New York Post photograph by Victor DeLucia © 1973, New York Post Corporation.

Nurses from the city's 19 municipal hospitals demonstrate during the dedication today of a $140 million medical center at Bellevue Hospital. The nurses are asking parity with salaries paid by private hospitals.

not for economic security but for the rewards gained through compassionate care for those in need. Unionization within hospitals would mean that doctors and nurses could be compared with truck drivers and miners.[13] Although the overall economy will not suffer when health care professionals go on strike, patient care will suffer, and the individual could suffer greatly.

The implications of unionizing traditional professions are obvious. The pride and satisfaction of performing a service will be lost among grievances, specifically defined tasks and strikes. The professional of today, however, has been influenced in the decision concerning unionization by rising inflation and living costs. Unionized blue collar workers as well as white collar employees who have already organized are keeping up with inflation through automatic pay raises, cost of living raises, and, in some cases, guaranteed annual income. The increases in salary of the health care professional, however, are met with the complaints of higher charges to the recipients of their professional care.[14]

To some professionals, union membership is no longer considered to be unethical or unprofessional. Instead, attention is turning toward the organization of a politically powerful organization that can best represent the needs of their profession. Already one can observe the bargaining victories of teachers, professors, and government unions. Nurses and other health care professionals no doubt have noticed the increasing activism and militancy displayed by doctors in a strike in New York City.[15]

Because the health care industry is virgin territory for labor unions, many different labor organizations are making serious efforts to unionize hospital employees. Coupled with the reasons mentioned above, it is a safe assumption that the efforts of labor unions will not go unrewarded. Therefore, it is no longer a question of whether a professional can belong to a union, but, to which union should the professional belong? It appears the prestige once afforded an ethical profession has given way to economic pressures and contractual agreements.

Unlike other industries, the health care complex offers its services to people who are in need of medical attention. Once admitted to a health care facility, the patients are dependent on the employees to deliver quality health care regardless of the costs involved. At present, there is much debate over how unionization of

health care professionals will ultimately effect the cost to patients.

NOTES

1. Dennis Dale Pointer, "Hospital Labor Relations Legislation: An Examination and Critique of Public Policy," *Hospital Progress* Vol. 54, No. 1 (January 1973): 71-75.
2. Dennis Dale Pointer, "How the Taft-Hartley Amendments Will Affect Health Care Facilities, Part 6," *Hospital Progress* Vol. 55, No. 10 (October 1974): 68-70.
3. Dennis Dale Pointer, "Hospital Labor Relations Legislation: An Examination and Critique of Public Policy," *Hospital Progress* Vol. 54, No. 1 (January 1973): 71-75.
4. *Central Dispensary and Emergency Hospital vs. NLRB,* 145 F.2d 852 (D.C. Cir. 1944) *cert. denied,* 342 U.S. 847, 65 Sup. Ct. 684 (1945).
5. *Ibid.*
6. Pointer, "Hospital Labor Relations Legislation: An Examination and Critique of Public Policy," *op. cit.*
7. *Ibid.*
8. *Ibid.*
9. *Ibid.*
10. *Ibid.*
11. S. P. Pepe and R. L. Murphy, "The NLRB Decisions on Appropriate Bargaining Units," *Hospital Progress* Vol. 56, No. 8 (August 1975): 43.
12. Dennis Dale Pointer, "How the 1974 Taft-Hartley Amendments Will Affect Health Care Facilities, Part 2," *Hospital Progress* Vol. 55, No. 11 (November 1974): 58-61.
13. Erwin S. Stanton, "Unions and the Professional Employee," *Hospital Progress* Vol. 54, No. 1 (January 1974): 58-59.
14. Vernon Coleman, "Can Anyone Be a Health Professional and A Trade Unionist?" *Nursing Mirror* Vol. 139, No. 9 (August 30, 1974): 41.
15. *Ibid.*

Chapter 3

"JAWS"
or
WHAT LABOR LAW CAN DO TO YOU IF GIVEN THE CHANCE

The purpose of the federal labor laws is to define and protect the rights of employees and employers, to encourage collective bargaining, and to eliminate certain practices on the part of labor and employers that are termed unfair labor practices. With its various amendments, the original Wagner Act is now called the National Labor Relations Act (NLRA).

The labor laws are administered by the National Labor Relations Board (NLRB) which consists of five members appointed by the president and confirmed by the Senate. The first NLRB took office in 1935, shortly after the Wagner Act was passed by Congress. The new board, on its own initiative, quickly established an administrative mechanism, which made it prosecutor, judge, and jury.

In the years that followed, public criticism of a system, which would allow a federal agency to sit as prosecutor, judge, and jury became intense. When Congress made major amendments to the Wagner Act by passage of the Labor-Management Relations Act of 1947, it established a unique system for the administration of the NLRB. In effect, Congress divided authority into two completely independent units, the board and the Office of the General Counsel.

The Office of the General Counsel was created to perform the preliminary functions of investigation and prosecution of unfair labor practice cases. The board was to restrict itself to deciding cases involving charges of unfair labor practices and determine representational questions that would come to it from the regional offices. Thus, the NLRB operates essentially as a court and makes decisions on the basis of a formal record.

The NLRB has two basic purposes. First, it defines and eliminates certain practices on the part of labor and employer that are deemed illegal under the act, called unfair labor practices. Second, it supervises and conducts secret ballot elections among employees to determine whether they want to be represented by a labor organization for purposes of collective bargaining. To accomplish these primary directives, the NLRB and the Office of the General Counsel act through forty-two regional and field offices located in major cities throughout the United States. If an employer or a labor union is charged with committing an unfair labor practice, the hearing and taking of evidence will be conducted at one of the regional offices located within the area where the union and employer are doing business, or where the unfair labor practice in question took place. Such a hearing is conducted before an administrative law judge from either Washington, D.C., or San Francisco, California, the home bases. However a hearing officer, usually an employee of the board's regional office, presides as the judge in both preelection and postelection representation hearings. In unfair labor practice hearings, the rules of evidence applicable in the District Courts of the United States are controlling "so far as practicable."[1] In representational hearings, the rules of evidence are not controlling because it is not considered as an adversary proceeding, merely a fact-finding inquiry.

REPRESENTATIONAL PROCEDURE

There are two basic ways in which a union can gain exclusive bargaining rights for a group of employees. The union can make formal demand to the employer for recognition based on authorization cards signed by a majority of the employees sought to be represented by the union. Since authorization cards are often obtained by the union through either outright misrepresentation or under circumstances when the employee does not fully understand the significance of his/her signature on authorization card, most employers do not recognize a union voluntarily based on such authorization cards. The second manner in which the union can become the bargaining agent is by filing a petition with the NLRB for a representation election. The board will require a thirty percent showing of interest from the union before processing such an election petition. The showing of interest is normally supplied by union authorization cards totaling at least thirty percent of all employees sought to be represented by the union.

Most unions will not file an election petition with the NLRB unless they get cards of more than fifty percent of the employees. Some unions even insist on sixty-five or seventy-five percent of the employees on signed authorization cards before they will file such a petition.

Upon receipt by the board of a petition for an election, a member of the board's staff then investigates the petition to determine: (1) if the unit that the union seeks to represent is appropriate under the act; (2) if there is a *bona fide* question concerning representation; (3) if the employer's operations affect commerce; (4) if an election would serve the interest and policies of the act; and (5) if the petitioner is a labor organization under the act. If all these criteria are met, the regional staff will attempt to persuade both the union and employer to agree to some form of consent election. If the parties refuse to enter into a form of consent election, a hearing is then held before a hearing officer of the regional office of the labor board. At this time both parties and the hearing officer can call and examine witnesses without being subject to the procedural rules followed in the federal district courts. After the hearing, the hearing officer submits a report to the regional director summarizing the issues and evidence, but containing no recommendations. The regional director then issues a report, either directing an election or dismissing the petition. If a difficult or novel issue of law is presented, the regional director can transfer the record to the board in Washington for a ruling. If an election has been ordered or consented to by management, a date is selected by the board for the election to be held. The employer is then required to furnish to the board at least two copies of the names and addresses of all employees eligible to vote in the election, one of such copies being sent to the union. Subsequently, an election is held, usually on the employer's premises.

EMPLOYER UNFAIR LABOR PRACTICES

The unfair labor practices of employers are listed in Section 8(a) of the act; those of labor organizations in Section 8(b). Section 8(a)(1) forbids an employer "to interfere with, restrain or coerce employees in the exercise of the rights guaranteed in Section 7." Section 7 of the act provides as follows:

> Employees shall have the right to self-organization, to form, join, or assist labor organizations, to bargain collectively through representatives of their own choosing, and to engage in other concerted activities for the purpose of collective bargaining or other mutual aid or protection, and shall also have the right to refrain from any or all of such activities except to the extent that such right may be affected by an agreement requiring membership in a labor organization as a condition of employment as authorized in Section 8(a)(3).

Some examples of employee rights protected by this section are as follows: (1) to join a union even if the union is not recognized by the employer; (2) to assist a union to organize the employees of an employer; (3) to form or attempt to form a union among the employees of the company; (4) to refrain from any activity in or on behalf of the union; and (5) to strike to secure better working conditions.

These rights guaranteed in Section 7 have been interpreted by the NLRB, with court approval, to mean that whatever specific unfair labor practice an employer commits, that action will automatically imply a violation of Section 8(a)(1). Therefore, whenever a violation of Section 8(a)(2), (3), (4), or (5) is committed by an employer, it is also a violation of Section 8(a)(1). In addition, a specific act or conduct by an employer could, of course, be an independent violation of Section 8(a)(1). Examples of such independent violations are as follows: (1) threatening to close down the hospital if a union should win the election; (2) questioning employees about their union activities or memberships in such circumstances as will tend to restrain or coerce the employee; (3) spying on union gatherings or meetings or pretending to spy on them; (4) threatening employees with loss of jobs or benefits if they should join or vote for a union; and (5) granting wage increases deliberately timed to discourage employees from forming or joining a union.

Section 8(a)(3) makes it an unfair labor practice for an employer to discriminate against employees "in regard to hire or tenure of employment for any term or condition of employment" for the purpose of encouraging or discouraging membership in a labor organization. Thus, the act makes it illegal for an employer to discriminate in employment because of an employee's union sentiments or his other group activity coming within the protection of the act. Discrimination within the meaning of this section would include such action as refusing to hire, discharging, demoting, assigning to a less desirable shift or job, or withholding benefits from any employee because of his union activities. As a supervisor engaged in supporting the hospital's position in a union organizational drive, these two sections of the labor act, 8(a)(1) and 8(a)(3), are those that should be of greatest concern. Indeed, the hospital would be unwise to violate the law intentionally. Instead, it should make every effort to train and instruct all supervisors and management personnel to insure that they do indeed refrain from committing a violation that could be construed as an unfair labor practice under the act.

EMPLOYER FREE SPEECH

An employer has a statutorily recognized right to communicate its views to the employees concerning unionization. Section 8(c) of the NLRA provides this free speech guarantee:

> the expressing of any views, arguments or opinions, or the dissemination thereof, whether in written, printed, graphic, or visual form, shall not constitute or be evidence of an unfair labor practice under any of the provisions of the sub-chapter if such expression contains no threat or reprisal or force or promise of benefit.[2]

This section applies equally to employers, employees, and labor organizations.

Thus the right of management to make known its views on unionization to its employees explicitly includes all communications, barring only those that threaten reprisals or promise benefits. Such threats or promises, to the extent that they coerce, restrain, or interfere with employee rights of self-organization, would constitute a violation of Section 8(a)(1).

INTERROGATING EMPLOYEES

The interrogation of employees by supervisors or management personnel is certainly one way of coercing employees from the exercise of their rights under the act. The right of management to question employees with respect to their union attitudes is very limited indeed. Do not ask employees what they think about the union or its representatives, how they intend to vote, or whether they are joining or already belong to a union. Moreover, supervisors should not ask an employee how he/she feels about the union or why there might be a need for a union at the hospital.

Some employees might give this or other information about the union to the supervisor or employer of their own accord. It is not unlawful to listen, as long as the supervisor or employer does not solicit the information or engage in questioning the employee in greater detail about the volunteered information.[3]

The hospital does have a right to wage an affirmative campaign on its behalf. It serves no legitimate reason or purpose, however, to interrogate employees concerning the union activity. Certainly, some employees will come out into the open wearing buttons or actively working as an in-house organizing committee on behalf of the union's organizational attempt. The hospital's role and duty is an affirmative sales campaign, *not* an interrogation of employees as to the identity of the prounion employees or an interrogation of the employees themselves about their union sentiments. It has been held in court cases to be coercive and in violation of the law for a supervisor to interrogate an employee about his/her union activities; to ask an employee if he is posing as a union plant; to inquire, shortly after a union supporter has been discharged, about conversations concerning the union; to ask an employee if he/she has signed a union authorization card; to ask if union officials have visited an employee's home at night; or to seek information about the identity of union supporters.

Surveillance

Any attempt on the part of the hospital or its supervisors to spy on the union activities of any employee or any acts of surveillance are considered inherently coercive and unlawful.[4]

Unlawful surveillance has been found in a variety of employer actions. The most blatant form of surveillance is having management personnel observe those employees attending union meetings, but even driving past a building in which a union meeting is underway has been held to constitute coercive surveillance. Similarly, writing down license plate numbers of employees attending union meetings is illegal. Statements suggesting that the major purpose and scope of the union's activities or that the identities of union supporters were known to management have both been held to justify charges of unlawful surveillance. In one case, even the implication that an employer would learn the identity of union supporters was held to violate the NLRA on the theory that the employer simultaneously had implied its expected information would be used for reprisal against union supporters.[5] Thus, even if no information is actually gathered by an employer or supervisor, merely creating an impression of surveillance can violate the act because of its intimidating effect.

An exception is again provided where an employee voluntarily communicates to his/her supervisor the details of union organizing activities. The courts generally have held that employers are not required to "close their ears" to voluntary employee statements about union activities, as long as no coercion could be shown or further interrogation of the employee was attempted by the supervisor.[6]

Threats and Loss of Benefits

It has been consistently held that an employer cannot deprive its employees of job benefits in an effort to coerce them into opposing union organization. Employers are also prohibited from threatening the employees with either the loss of a job benefit or benefits or any other job-related consequences as retaliation for union support. This clearly constitutes a violation of Section 8(a)(1), inhibiting employees from their protected rights to self-organization.

A single incident resulting in a threat of a lost benefit can be sufficient grounds to set aside an election if the hospital wins. The hospital, therefore, has to be careful that it makes no threats about the loss of any employee benefit either directly or indirectly. Examples of direct threats of loss of benefits include such things as ending the practice of giving employees Christmas bonuses, ending the practice of periodic wage increases, revoking permission for employees to take advantage of discounts, stopping the occasional practice of handing out wage checks in advance of payday, eliminating employee rest periods, and discontinuing direct loans to employees. Indirect threats of loss of benefits occur whenever a hospital withholds any benefit from union members or supporters while awarding the same benefits to nonunion employees. Examples of this practice have included the awarding of additional holidays to all employees except those in the voting unit.[7]

Threats of employer retaliation concerning employment are certainly as coercive as the actual deprivation of benefits; they, accordingly, are illegal. No employee can be threatened with discharge or any form of job discrimination for joining or supporting a union, nor can he be told that the hospital will close if the union is successful.[8]

Violations of Section 8(a)(1) have been found in circumstances such as: statements that new work rules were put into effect because of employees' union support, in suggestions that employees could sign a petition that they did not wish to be represented by a union, in threats of adverse economic consequences, in warnings that unionization would cause the discharge of nonproductive workers, in statements that union members would not be hired by other employers, and in general threats of discharge and layoff.

The hospital certainly should take every precaution to see that threats are not made to the employees. Employees have the unquestionable right to make the selection for or against the union without fear of intimidation, coercion, or threats from the union side, or from the hospital's side. The hospital should endeavor to insure that no threatening conduct of any kind, even by implication, is stated to an employee. For example, do not state that it will serve no useful purpose to vote for the union because the employees could lose benefits that have been gratitutiously bestowed upon them.

Promise or Grant of Benefits

As soon as the hospital is charged with actual knowledge that a unionization attempt is being made, it is prohibited from granting or promising any additional benefits. This prohibition seems reasonable; management naturally might want to react to a union organization attempt by granting an increase in benefits or wages to persuade employees that they will receive satisfactory wages and conditions without assistance of any union. The law clearly provides that an employer can neither promise nor grant employees any new benefits in an attempt to defeat the union organization effort. Thus it has been held illegal to grant current or retroactive pay raises, any improved vacation benefits, scheduling changes, or additional Christmas bonuses. All such actions taken after the hospital has notice of the union organizational attempt are illegal. Prior to such knowledge of the organizational attempt, the employer can grant whatever benefit its enlightened self-interest dictates.

Similarly, the employer has little latitude in pledging or promising benefits once a union organizational campaign has commenced. The most frequent promises held to be violations of employee rights are those that pledge wage increases, improved insurance benefits, employee credit unions, changes in vacations or sick benefits, or a longer duration of employment for temporary workers.

NOTES

1. 29 U.S.C. § 160(b) (1970).
2. 29 U.S.C. § 158(c) (1970).
3. *Jeffco Mfg. Co.*, 211 N.L.R.B. no. 17 (1974).
4. *Hendrix Mfg. Co. vs. N.L.R.B.*, 321 F.2d 100, 100-105 Note 7 (5th Cir. 1963); *NLRB vs. Collins and Aikman Corporation*, 146 F.2d 454 (4th Cir. 1944).
5. *NLRB vs. Finesilver Mfg. Co.*, 400 F.2d 644, 646 (5th Cir. 1968).
6. *NLRB vs. Atkins Saw Division, Nicholson File Co.*, 39 F.2d 907, 910 (5th Cir. 1968).
7. *NLRB vs. Great A&P Tea Company*, 409 F.2d 296, 297-298 (5th Cir. 1969).
8. *Parke Coal Co.*, 219 N.L.R.B. no. 50 (1975).

Sample Union
Flyers and Handbills

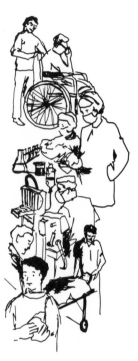

Whether you're a nurse, an aide or an orderly, a dietary, laundry or custodial worker, a clerk or a technician, the work you do at your hospital helps sick people get well. That's what you do—you help people.

We help people, too. We're the Service Employees International Union, the largest union of hospital workers in the United States. Of our one-half million members, 200,000 work in the health care industry, holding down jobs just like yours.

For more than 50 years we've made it our job to help people with your job. We're the biggest health care workers' union in the country, and we're the best.

SEIU's Local 250 in Northern California is the biggest local union of hospital workers in the country. Local 144 in New York, Local 399 in Los Angeles and Local 79 in Detroit each represent thousands of hospital workers. And so do scores of others SEIU local unions in places like Portland, Seattle, Denver, Chicago, St. Louis and elsewhere.

SEIU represents hospital workers in smaller towns, too. Towns like Burlington, Iowa and Paducah, Kentucky, just to name a couple. In big cities and small towns alike, health care workers rely on SEIU to help them win bigger paychecks and better benefits.

Two hundred thousand health care workers have found that there's a union that cares—Service Employees International Union, one of the ten biggest unions in the AFL-CIO. We're the biggest union in the field, and the best. Just ask our 200,000 members—they know better than anybody.

(Tear off at dotted line and mail. No stamp necessary.)

Hospital Workers Organizing Committee
Service Employees International Union, AFL-CIO

Yes, I'd like to know more about how SEIU can help me get higher wages and better benefits.
☐ Please send me more information.
☐ I will help form an SEIU Committee. Please have a hospital union representative contact me.

My name is: . . . .

My address is: . . . . Phone . . . .

I work at: . . . .

Address: . . . .

Signed: . . . .

How's it going?

No problems with your supervisor? No fear of unjust firing? Never a bad moment getting the correct holiday and vacation leave? Courtesy and respect from management? Never had any problems?

If the answers are yes, you're doing pretty well. But the odds are that somewhere down the line you've gotten a bad deal, and haven't been able to do a thing about it. You were in the right, they were in the wrong, but you lost out anyway.

That doesn't have to happen. Union contracts provide a system by which problems can be worked out—fairly. In most contracts, if you and your union representative can't arrive at a fair solution with management, a third party—an "arbitrator"—is called in to resolve it. Under the contract, management has to go along with the arbitrator's ruling, even if they don't like it. It's the law.

Just about every one of SEIU's 200,000 health care industry members is protected by a grievance procedure. They don't have to worry about being fired just because their supervisor got up on the wrong side of the bed. They've got some protection.

You can have that protection, too. An SEIU-negotiated union contract can give it to you. Millions of Americans go to work every day without having to worry about having their jobs at the end of the day because of a boss's whim: these workers know that their union contract gives them basic protections. With SEIU, these protections could be yours, too.

If you are interested in learning more about what SEIU can do for the people where you work, mail the attached card.

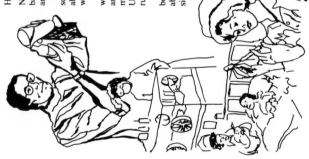

(Tear off at dotted line and mail. No stamp necessary.)

Hospital Workers Organizing Committee
Service Employees International Union, AFL-CIO

Yes, I'd like to know more about how SEIU can help me get higher wages and better benefits.
☐ Please send me more information.
☐ I will help form an SEIU Committee. Please have a hospital union representative contact me.

My name is: ....

My address is: .... Phone ....

I work at: ....

Address: ....

Signed: ....

ARE YOU GOING TO VOTE FOR THE UNION ?

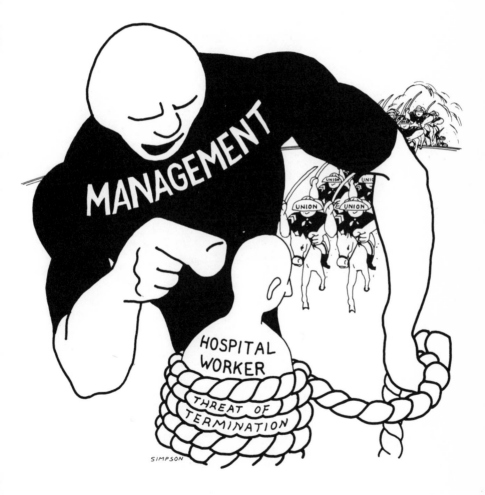

Chapter 4

WHO'S WHO AMONG SUPERVISORS
or
MAKE ROOM FOR THE BOARD

The problem really begins with the question, just what is a supervisor under the National Labor Relations Act (NLRA)? Good question. However the answer is not, and cannot, be clearly stated. The National Labor Relations Board (NLRB) has refused to issue clear guidelines or definitions applicable to all supervisors. Instead, the board has stated repeatedly that a particular individual's supervisory status is to be determined on a case-by-case basis depending on the particular facts involved.

Although many have criticized the board as inconsistent and unpredictable on supervisory questions, it should be noted that, with all possible variations of supervisors, it is a difficult problem. So the board looks at the reality of the actual duties, responsibilities, and job functions of the particular supervisor in question. To do this, testimony is taken from employees, the supervisor involved, and his/her supervisors and/or department heads to establish the actual day by day facts of each supervisor's particular job at the hospital.

The act itself defines a supervisor in Section 2(11) as follows:

The term "supervisor" means any individual having authority, in the interest of the employer, to hire, transfer, suspend, lay off, recall, promote, discharge, assign, reward, or discipline other employees, or responsibly to direct them, or to adjust their grievances, or effectively to recommend such action, if in connection with the foregoing the exercise of such authority is not of a merely routine or clerical nature, but requires the use of independent judgment.[1]

The board and courts, however, have put highly technical and legalistic considerations on the numerous factual situations presented, so the definition itself is only the beginning point in determining supervisory status. The fact that other federal or state laws or agencies consider someone to be a supervisor, or exempt as an executive or part of management, is meaningless in resolving Section 2(11) supervisory status under the act. Consequently, this is a new and different issue that can be resolved only by reference to the NLRA and the decisions issued under that law.

In many cases supervisory status is so clear that neither the union nor the labor board will question it. Department heads and the administrator and his/her staff generally fall into this category. The real gray area is line supervisors or working supervisors. In many cases, line supervisors in housekeeping and dietary departments are in a questionable position in light of the Section 2(11) definition. Similarly among nurses, charge nurses or head nurses present problems.

AN EDUCATED GUESS

Some of these issues have been presented recently to the board. However, even if one were to read all the board's decisions, the inconsistencies and confusion would still be evident. So how does anyone ever determine the questionable supervisory issues in a hospital? By investigating the facts and actual day to day functions, in much the same way the board does, one can make an educated guess.

The hospital has to make that educated guess early in the union's organizing drive, and it is an important one. It has to be made early because the hospital must do what is allowed—hold meetings to train supervisors to respond to the union's organizational drive. It is an unfair labor practice under the act for a hospital to solicit the direct involvement of an employee in its campaign against the union. Since early action by a hospital's supervisors can prevent the union from getting sufficient employees to sign authorization cards and secure an NLRB supervised election, the question of who is a supervisor is very impor-

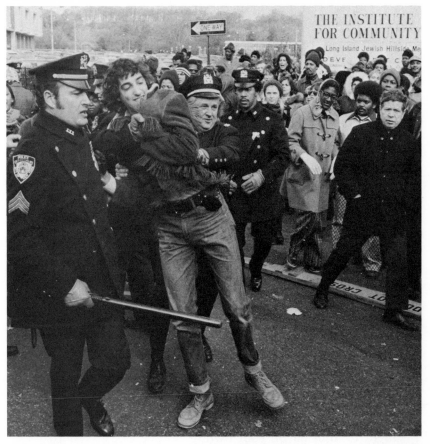

New York Daily News. Reprinted with permission.

Cops remove a picket from entrance to Long Island Jewish Hospital, New Hyde Park, L.I.

tant. Even once the cards are signed, the supervisors can still work in the campaign to convince employees to vote against the union at the NLRB supervised election. Moreover, supervisors are not a part of any successful union bargaining contract or strike situation.

The hospital itself should take definite steps before any union actively begins by defining its Section 2(11) supervisors under the NLRA. To properly do so requires an honest consideration, and some serious decisions about the various functions that a specific job may have.

TESTING YOUR GUESS

Once it is realized that making a determination about certain hospital supervisors and their Section 2(11) status under the act is a thorny problem, the following self-examination test is recommended only as an assistance. The only preexamination instructions offered are to think carefully before answering each question with a simple yes or no. Before writing down the answer for a particular question, consider what you would offer in documentation or explanation to the hospital's labor attorney. It is the attorney who must present such evidence at a hearing to prove your answer. Such evidence can be oral testimony, from yourself or from some of the employees under your supervision or that of your supervisors. Past practice and written evidence also play important roles in establishing that you are a supervisor.

With these few points in mind, answer these questions carefully:

Question	Possible Points for Yes
1. Do you hire new employees?	10
2. Do you transfer employees from one department to another on your own?	10
3. Do you discipline employees? (e.g., issue written warnings, give suspensions)	10
4. Do you lay off employees?	10
5. Do you recall employees?	10
6. a. Do you promote employees?	10
b. Are your recommendations for promotion, including merit increases, upgrading, or job-related settlements generally accepted or given considerable weight by your supervisors in determining action to be taken? (as opposed to the mere privilege of giving recommendations)	10

7. Do you discharge employees? 10

8. Do you assign employees to work on your own authority? (as opposed merely to relaying orders or assigning from written work schedules) 9

9. Do you enforce hospital rules against employees or adjust grievances for employees on your own? 8

10. Do you direct employees in their work? (as opposed to relaying orders and directions of others) 8

11. Do you make up layoff lists that are followed without veto from higher authority? 8

12. Do you recommend to accept or reject a supplier? 8

13. Do you "okay" late or early punching out by others? (e.g., excuse further attendance during work hours) 5

14. Do you have ten or more employees under your supervision? 5

15. Do you occasionally take the place of an admitted supervisor when the latter is absent? 4

16. Do you receive greater vacation, holiday, sick leave, insurance, pension, or other benefits than employees under your supervision? 4

17. Do you attend meetings, training workshops, or seminars held for hospital supervisors? 4

18. Are you one of several consulted on layoffs? 4

19. Do you pledge the credit of the hospital for purchases? 3

20. Do you work overtime or extra shifts without added compensation? 3

21. If paid hourly, is your wage rate fifty cents or more above the highest hourly rated employee under you? 3

22. Do you have the title of supervisor or manager, and are your employees aware of it?   3

23. Do you have and exercise the authority to change work schedules?   2

24. Do you have the authority to decide and assign overtime to your employees?   2

25. Are you paid a salary while all employees under you are paid hourly?   2

26. Are you designated on the payroll, personnel, or hospital records as a supervisor?   2

27. Do you wear clothes or a uniform different from other employees?   1

28. Do you instruct or train new employees on job duties?   1

29. Do you keep time and attendance records?   1

30. Are you the only person with apparent authority present on a given shift or in a separate department?   1

31. Do you use parking lots, dining rooms, etc. reserved for management or supervisors?   1

TOTAL _____

Date Test Taken _____ day of _____, 19____

Upon completion of the test, if your total points exceed twenty you most likely will be held to be a supervisor under Section 2(11) of the act. The more points over twenty, the more likely this result will occur. However, if you only have ten to twenty points, you are in the gray area or "coin-flipping" situation. Only by an in-depth study and careful consideration of your job can a reasonable prediction be made. If you have less than ten total points, you most probably are not a supervisor under Section 2(11).

NOTES

1. Vernon Coleman, "Can Anyone Be a Health Professional and a Trade Unionist?" *Nursing Mirror* Vol. 139 (August 30, 1974): 41.

Chapter 5

THE METHOD BEHIND THE MADNESS
or
KNOW YOUR ADVERSARY

The five largest and most active unions in the health care field are the American Federation of State, County, and Municipal Employees; the Service Employees National Union; and the National Union of Hospital and Health Care Employees (all three are affiliates of the AFL-CIO); the Teamsters; and the American Nurses Association (ANA). In addition, there are other professional associations similar to the ANA that are actually quasi-unions, since they express the views of the members and are making demands for collective bargaining rights. At their convention in June 1974, in San Francisco, the ANA passed an emergency resolution supporting the strike of 4,000 nurses in the area.[1]

The unions are more than eager to provide the necessary help in organizing labor in hospitals. The massive numbers employed represent considerable dues income to unions. In the authors' immediate Houston area, union representatives have distributed handbills to over thirty hospitals and have held National Labor Relations Board (NLRB) scheduled elections at seven health care facilities within only a six-month period. Unions are dedicated to win the war against management.

THE BARGAINING ELECTION PROCESS—AN OVERVIEW

The bargaining unit determination and election processes are set in motion after a petition for an election has been filed with the NLRB. This petition can be filed by an employee, a group of employees, or an individual of a labor organization acting on behalf of the employees. The NLRB requires such petition to be supported by a showing of interest from at least thirty percent of the employees sought to be represented. Upon receipt of the petition, the NLRB conducts an investigation and may hold a hearing to determine:

1. if jurisdiction can be asserted under the act,
2. whether sufficient interest on the part of the employees has been demonstrated,
3. if an election is being sought in an appropriate unit,
4. whether the union named in the petition is qualified to participate in an election, and
5. whether there are any existing barriers against holding an election. [2]

Sometimes elections are the result of an agreement between the employer and union representative. If neither can agree to have the election, the NLRB has the authority to order a representation hearing and order an election to be conducted under the direction of the NLRB regional office. In such an election several guidelines are followed.

1. More than one union may appear on the ballot.
2. Eligibility to vote is determined by a previous payroll roster of the employees.
3. The election is usually held on the employee's premises in an area easily accessible by employees and at a time opportune for the employees.
4. The NLRB supplies the ballot upon which is listed all options, i.e., choice between union(s) and no union.
5. Each party may have observers at the polling place and challenge any employee's right to vote.
6. Ballots are tabulated by the NLRB at the conclusion of the voting period, in the presence of observers. A majority of the votes cast are required for union representation. If more than one union was on the ballot and the vote was split, a runoff election would be held.
7. Within five days of the announcement of results, both parties can challenge the election on the grounds that: (a) the manner in which the election was held was illegal; (b) the employer or union intimidated employees; (c) false promises

or misrepresentations were made; and (d) reproductions of the official ballot were misused as campaign literature.[3]

Should the union lose the election, the union must wait at least one year before petitioning for another election in the same unit.

Because the health care industry is relatively new territory for unions, the recent expansion in collective bargaining agencies in hospitals is expected to continue in even greater proportions. It is clear that unions have one terrific advantage over hospital management—experience. Due to their experience, unions will know exactly how to approach hospital employees, persuade them to unionize, and utilize available alternatives in the event of unfair labor practices. Management, on the other hand, will be forced to learn from its mistakes, mistakes which could well be hazardous to the hospital.

THE UNION ORGANIZER

Good union organizers are active practicing "psychologists." The organizers' expertise is human relations; and in such a field, unorganized working men and women are the raw materials to be refined by the professional union organizer through group action.

Basic Tools of a Union Organizer

Three primary personality tools make a successful union organizer, and a good practitioner usually is amply talented in all three. First, he/she needs a native quality and capacity to like people. This is more than just back slapping, telling jokes, and having beer with the boys. A union organizer is a warm, gentle, outgoing person who communicates and relates effectively to all types of people.

Second, he/she needs the ability to adapt to the immediate surroundings. A union organizer, as the lizard which changes colors, must adapt to his immediate surroundings and not feel superior or out of place among any group of employees. He has the tendency to warm up to people very quickly, usually within ten or fifteen minutes after meeting a new prospect.

Finally, patience with people is his *forte*. A union organizer is a patient person. Nonunion employees are rarely completely sold on the idea of union organizing or unionism in the first discussion. The union organizer realizes this and considers it an ongoing effort to sign up or convince all employees about the values of unionism and collective action.

Union Organizing Strategy

Regardless of the union, the organizer has one primary advantage over his opposition in health care administration: he is a trained fighter. He has been to war many times and has lost some, but won many. The majority of union organizers have come up through the ranks. It is a grave error to underrate the casual dress and slang language. Beneath the innocent or unpolished exterior lurks the mind of a well-organized trained soldier.

The bargaining units of the AFL-CIO and the Teamsters represent the most sophisticated union threat. The ANA and other such associations are still fighting among themselves as to the degree of "union" they want to be. They lack the experience of the older, more established unions; and they lack the track record.

Each union carefully trains its organizers and usually has a detailed guidebook to cover almost every conceivable situation. It is worthwhile to look at the union adversary and determine the specific campaign strategy being used in your facility. Union organizing attempts primarily incorporate one or more of three steps.

STEP 1:   The Hospital Survey. Background information is a necessary part of any campaign. Unless the organizer has a thorough understanding of the hospital, its policies, its key people, its problems, etc., a formalized strategy cannot be developed. Consequently, the first step is to do a "target" survey.

Initially, the organizer spends several hours simply observing the facility, talking to cafeteria employees, workers in housekeeping, nurses, and so on. From such conversations the organizer attempts to determine the number of employees per shift; employee breakdown by sex, age, race, etc.; what eating and drinking facilities are nearby; available transportation facilities for the employees; and special problems the facility might face.

The second part of a survey involves establishing contact with the existing labor movement in the community. Here the organizer determines the labor position of the mass media; the labor history of the organization; names of employees who are active in community work such as churches, civic groups, and politics (these persons often make good initial contacts); names of former employees who belonged to a union; a general idea of wages, conditions, and problems; community relations with the target facility; community reaction to organized labor; and meeting dates and places for local union groups.

STEP 2:   Selecting the Employee Leaders. Having completed his initial survey of the facility, the organizer is now ready to make his first contact with the employees of the health care facility. Most union organizers are primarily interested in finding the employee who is respected by his/her fellow workers and who has informal influence within the health care facility. These are the workers that the organizer will depend on for "internal leadership" and information about the specific problems and complaints of the employees.

The labor organizers court potential internal leaders. The benefits of the union are explained, and an attempt is made to build up the trust of the leaders. The organizers try to get leaders for every faction within the organization; for the women, the men, the minority groups, etc. They create committees and encourage mass participation.

The importance of in-house employee organizers cannot be over emphasized. As a Teamsters' union organizing training manual states,

> . . .the real job of organization will take place inside the plant or shop from day to day and hour to hour under the nose of the foreman or supervisors. The organizer can only implement and give general directions from the outside. The basic job of bringing people together for the common cause can only be successfully done by the group itself

under the day to day leadership of key contacts within the plant.[4]

STEP 3:   Showing the Union Presence. In Step 3 the union will begin actively to distribute handbills and/or begin seeking authorization card signatures for the purpose of forcing an election. The purpose of this first handout distribution is little more than to show union presence. Such leaflets tend to be general in nature and are usually prepared by the union's international or national office.

Once the "internal leaders" begin bringing the organizer the signed union authorization cards, the organizer dramatically steps up the campaign by seeking the trouble spots, evaluating internal leadership, determining the area in which to build additional support, and determining the best areas for the key supporters within the health care facility.

Demand for Recognition

Early in a campaign the union usually will send a telegram, letter, or even the organizer in person demanding recognition as the official bargaining unit for the health care employees. This demand for recognition usually asserts that:

1. the union has been officially designated as the exclusive bargaining agent by the majority of employees in the bargaining unit,
2. the union is prepared to begin immediate bargaining with management,
3. the union is prepared to present its authorization cards to management or to a third party to validate its claim of majority representation, and
4. the employer should beware of violating its "employees" statutory rights guaranteed under the National Labor Relations Act.

The purpose in sending this demand is to seek voluntary recognition without an election. Failing that, the demand is reflected in the official petition for an election filed to initiate the National

Labor Relations Board's election procedures. Health care supervisors should be aware of the dangers in this demand for recognition, however.

An unwary administrator can accept the demand without question (out of fear or uncertainty) and become straddled with a union. Labor counsel should be consulted first. Usually, labor counsel will send a standard letter to the union stating that the hospital doubts that the union represents an uncoerced majority of employees; the hospital believes that the best method for determining the true wishes of the employees is through the secret ballot; the hospital has no knowledge of the method by which the union solicited authorization cards and, thus, cannot accept their validity (management should be certain not to examine the cards or to agree to a third party examination); and the hospital recommends that the union file an election petition with the NLRB, which has jurisdiction over such activities.

Union Authorization Card

The typical union authorization card simply authorizes the union to act as an employee's agent for purposes of collective bargaining with the hospital.

In addition, the card serves four other important purposes. The first one is to satisfy the NLRB's thirty percent showing of interest requirement. In other words, the union must obtain a thirty percent show of interest by signed authorization cards or employees' signatures on a petition to file with the NLRB to hold a secret ballot election (conducted by the NLRB).

Second, the authorization cards are usually a reliable barometer of the employee sentiment within the hospital. Third, authorization cards are useful for an internal purpose. Union organizers are judged by their productivity, measured by the number of new authorization cards that the union organizer reports to his superiors. This, of course, makes it tempting to the union organizer to forge or persuade employees to sign cards without regard to the employees' real interest in the union.

Fourth, a hospital can be ordered by the NLRB to bargain with the union, even if the union lost the election. This can happen if fifty percent or more of the employees have signed authorization cards *and* the employer/hospital commits serious unfair labor practices, which tend to preclude the possibility of conducting a second election.

Having failed to get management to agree voluntarily to collective bargaining, it now becomes necessary to carry the campaign toward an election. The majority of effort is spent on encouraging those that signed the cards to actually vote for the union. Inside the health care facility the prounion employees try to persuade the other employees to support the effort. Participation is the key word in a union organizing attempt. The organizers create all types of committees (whether they need them or not). A union training manual states, "there is always room for more help in a campaign. Participation demonstrates to the individual worker that he/she is helping to build his or her union and to generate enthusiasm for the union within the plant."[5] Committees include, but are not limited to:

1. membership (accumulate potential members, names, groups);
2. publicity (to discuss union information within the facility);
3. distribution (mimeographing, handing out pamphlets, maintaining mailing lists, etc.);
4. strategy (works with organizer in developing tactics and strategies for the campaign effort); and
5. community (to explain the need for the union to the community and to try to get its support).

Another primary purpose for getting as many inside workers as possible on committees is to prevent management from claiming that the union activity is the result of "outside agititation," or to protect from the attack that it is the work of "a minority of disgruntled employees."

OTHER MAJOR UNION TACTICS

Meetings

The major reason for union meetings is to achieve a large turnout, thereby demonstrating solidarity, strength, and enthusiasm and getting the union's message over to the greatest number of employees at the same time.

Because publicly announced meetings always run the risk of being poorly attended, the early meetings are scheduled mostly by word of mouth. Once scheduled, the organizer spares *no* effort in filling the meeting hall. Beer, drinks, etc. are usually the fare. The ploy is "come on over and just hear what we have to say. Even if you don't like it, you can have all the free beer you can drink." Once there, the employee tends to think all the others in attendance are prounion.

The meetings are carefully *staged* with speakers instructed to keep their talks brief and with time always scheduled for a question and answer period. Union promises are seldom specific, they tend to be more general with an emphasis on "we can do it if we stick together." Such meetings always have "good" contracts from other health care institutions available to show "what can be done." Sometimes these contracts stretch the imagination. The authors once discovered that a 500 bed hospital in a high rent area of Philadelphia (recently organized) was the "contract" model used by the union organizing a poor 150-bed unit in a low cost of living area in Texas. The employees were impressed that wages were thirty percent higher. Of course, investigation later showed that the cost of living in Philadelphia was higher by about the same percent.

Before the meeting adjourns, the organizer attempts to secure additional authorization cards. Employees who will take cards and distribute them are encouraged to do so. The organizer notes each member there and tries to schedule a house call as he is introducing himself.

House Call

The house call is considered to be one of the most important tactics in a union organizing campaign. The employee is visited at home, and it is in this environment that the generalities accompanying a union campaign can be dropped. The individual's complaints and problems can be discussed and an explanation given on "how the union can help." It is here that more specific promises can be made. The union member making the house call at-

tempts to get the relationship on a buddy basis . . . making it us
(union and employee) against big, old, powerful-autocratic them
(management).

Telephone Campaign

In large bargaining units it becomes necessary to limit house
calls somewhat and become more dependent upon the telephone.
Teams of volunteer callers are set up, and the routine follows the
same essential pattern as the house call.

Publicity

Publicity is used as a weapon in every organizing campaign.
Publicity efforts include handbills, advertising in the mass media,
news releases, union movies, mail sent to homes of the employees,
and other such material.

In most of the publicity, the emphasis is on the emotional appeal. Use of such words as dignity, security, justice, fear, threats,
self respect, etc., are often used.

Union handbills all have three points in common: (1) they have
some type of eye-appealing attraction (usually a cartoon) to get
attention; (2) one or (at most) two issues are discussed briefly;
and (3) a method of settling the problem (vote union!) is at the
bottom of the handout. Sometimes a cartoon can be redrawn and
used by management against the union with great success. In one
campaign the authors were waging, the union distributed an anti-
management handbill. Pictured on the front was a poor hobo with
his hand out for a dime saying, "and management said I didn't
need a union." The authors redrew this by adding a flag (held up
by the hand sticking out) which read "on strike." Needless to say,
the union did not appreciate the changes in its own handout.

Warning the Employees

Warning the employees is a favorite ploy of unions. They seek
to tell in advance what the hospital will say and do. Obviously,
having so much experience (health care management is at a disadvantage here), the union organizer knows specifically what the

hospital will say and do; that they will become nicer, will start stating the reasons for employees not needing a union, and so on. Consequently, when the hospital begins to take such predictable measures, the employee is lead to think, "Well, if the union was right about this, it must be right about other things." The key to management, here, is to do the unexpected, to take the offense, and to tell the employees what the union is going to do.

ELECTION DAY ACTIVITY

The NLRB will set aside any election if an election speech is made to massed assemblies of employees on hospital time within twenty-four hours before the scheduled time for starting the election. The union, however, still works hard on the last day. They are still out trying to "talk up" the union with employees on a one-to-one basis. They also work to turn out the vote. A committee is usually appointed to watch who has and has not voted. Phone calls are made, and others provide cars for those needing transportation to the polls.

If the union organizer feels (usually the day before the election) that the outcome of the vote will be close or that he might lose, he will increase his challenge of certain voters (those most likely to vote nonunion). Such votes are then placed in a separate envelope and are counted separately (and at a later time). The result of such a ploy is to throw the election outcome into uncertainty. This has certain advantages when the organizer is working to unionize several institutions and does not want a loss on the record for the union at that particular time.

AFTER THE ELECTION

If management wins by a large vote, it is unlikely that the union will file objections to the election. If the majority vote is narrow, however, then objections are almost a certainty.

The union will usually contrive a story for the employee supporters if they lose—that management used unfair labor practices, fired employees for union activities, and so on. Again, the purpose is to make the election loss appear more as a strategic withdrawal than an actual defeat.

WHAT A UNION VICTORY MEANS TO YOU

If the union wins the election and negotiates a collective bargaining agreement with your hospital, you are the one who will have to deal with the union on a daily basis, with the union steward, with the grievances and arbitrations, with the complaints, with the slowdowns, and with the harassment.

As a supervisor your main function is working with employees and making daily decisions about each one. These decisions can involve discipline, discharge, promotion, overtime, work schedules, transfers, job assignments, and any number of others. The point is that in a nonunion status these decisions remain yours and the hospital's and should relate to the overall purpose of a hospital: quality patient care. With a union, however, your actions in all these areas can be the subject of union challenge. To make matters worse, the union steward, an employee picked by the union, is most often an employee with whom you are least able to get along on a day to day basis. Specifically, you will find your management rights drastically limited in the four areas.

Discipline. A union will severely curtail your authority to discipline employees. With a union contract, displinary actions such as reprimands or suspensions must first be taken up with the union steward, and perhaps even the business representative of the union. At the time of your action the union will examine your management record for any pattern of employee discrimination or favoritism. Additionally, the union makes discharge, as a form of discipline, a near impossibility.

Promotions. Management authority to promote employees based on job competence and ability to learn is virtually eliminated. Seniority or time in service becomes the main and sometimes only yardstick for measuring an employee's eligibility for performance. In fact, the hospital's refusal to promote a long service employee must have a detailed written justification.

Work scheduling and assignments. The scheduling of work and the assignment of job tasks is vastly complicated by union presence. Job descriptions must be followed to the letter. No task can be given an employee without that task being presented in a formally prepared and negotiated job description. For example, a delivery truck, too large to fit an unloading ramp, recently pulled up to a major unionized hospital in New York City containing badly needed beds for an intensive care unit. Because of its size the truck had to be located away from receiving. The receiving department employees refused to work in other than their designated area, and housekeeping personnel refused to unload because it was not in their job description. Consequently, the unloading of twenty electric beds and all components was accomplished by the supervisors from various departments, includ-

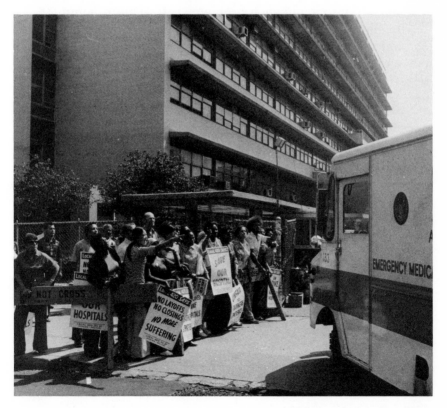

New York Daily News. Reprinted with permission.

Coney Island Hospital: Municipal hospital workers behind police barricade jeer arriving ambulance. Ambulance drivers worked under prestrike agreement.

ing housekeeping, maintenance, nursing, personnel, and administration.

Strikes, walkouts, slowdowns, and sick-ins. The stoppage of work in a health care facility represents a real threat to management and the welfare of patients whom the hospital is dedicated to protect. Strikes, walkouts, slowdowns, or other types of work stoppages can be called by the union for just reason, little reason, or no reason at all—the latter two seeming to be the most predominant. Should a strike occur, the health care facility is literally shut down. The simple delivery of a unit of blood from an outside source becomes a major problem. Violence and sabotage can happen, as evidenced by health care union strikes in such states as New York, Illinois, and California—to name only a few. The only way to avoid such problems is to remain nonunion.

The purpose of this chapter has been to demonstrate the dynamics of the adversary in a war, which, for nicety, is called a labor union campaign. Obviously, it is to the hospital's best interest to know the tactics of its adversary before developing its own campaign to win the war.

NOTES

1. Dennis Dale Pointer, "How the 1974 Taft-Hartley Amendments Will Affect Health Care Facilities, Part 1," *Hospital Progress* Vol. 55, No. 10 (October 1974): 68-70.
2. *Ibid.*
3. *Ibid.*
4. "Some Notes For Trade Union Organizers" (Central States Conference on Teamsters, International Brotherhood of Teamsters, 19).
5. *Guidebook for Union Organizers* (AFL-CIO, Industrial Union Department, 1972).

Sample Union
Flyers and Handbills

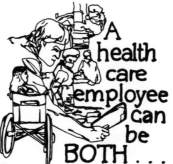

● **DEDICATED**
   TO YOUR JOB

Dedication to your job
is an obvious
necessity!

If you weren't
dedicated, you would
not be in the health
care profession!

You care -- that's why you
do what you do! You are dedicated
to do your job

A **health care employee can be BOTH** ...

● **RESPONSIBLE**
   TO YOURSELF

RESPONSIBILITY to
yourself is obviously just
as important!

You must look out for your
own needs -- your own goals
in life in in your work!

You must be responsible for
the welfare of yourself
and your family

If you want to be both DEDICATED TO YOUR JOB AND RESPONSIBLE
TO YOURSELF, then perhaps you should take a serious look at
one of the fastest growing labor organizations for health
care employees, the Hospital and Nursing Home Division of
Retail Clerks International Association.

Throughout the United States, thousands of employees in nursing
homes and hospitals have decided that they no longer wish to be
"second class" citizens when it comes to wages, hours, and
conditions of work. They have seen how the cost of living has
skyrocketed while their pay remains low -- and they have done
something about it!

The Federal Law now protects your right to form a Union and
your right to have a union contract without fear of coercive or
discriminatory action being taken against you by your administrator or supervisors.

Attached you will find a postage-paid, pre-addressed authorization
card. By filling out and mailing this card, you are taking the
first step toward having the true job security and increased
benefits of a union contract that so many of your fellow employees
in nursing homes and hospitals already enjoy.

These cards are confidential and WILL NOT BE SEEN by your
employer!

Fill out and mail your card today! If you want more information
please call 694-5541.

HOSPITAL & NURSING HOME
DIVISION

RETAIL CLERKS UNION, LOCAL NO. 455 AFL-CIO
4615 NORTH FREEWAY, SUITE 300
HOUSTON, TEXAS   77022

CLERICAL WORKERS ARE THE UNSUNG HEROINES OF EVERY HOSPITAL

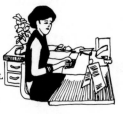

Usually tucked away behind the scenes, its the clerical workers who do all of the paperwork without which any hospital would shut down in confusion inside of 24 hours.

From the accounting office to the switchboard to the supply section, these "paper slingers" keep the administrative wheels turning; they keep the cash flowing and the mails moving. They are the oil that keeps the health machine in working order.

Without a competent, experienced clerical force, any hospital would be in big trouble--in fact, it would be out of business. But while that's the case, hospital administrators will be the last to admit it. Because if they did, hospital clerical workers would be enjoying better wages and benefits than they do today.

It's sad but true that Hospital wages are low--very low. And hospital clerical employees sufer as much, if not more, than all other hospital employees. Without a union, hospital clerical workers, just like the other employees in the hospital, just don't get a fair shake.

There's a union in town that can help make things a lot better. It's the union that represents more health care clerical workers than any other union in the country. The name is Service Employees International Union, AFL-CIO--a union of more than one-half million members, with 200,00 of those members working in the health care industry.

SEIU local unions from New York to California and virtually all points in between have negotiated collective bargaining agreements that bring recognition to hospital clerical workers--recognition in terms of money, in terms of benefits like vacations, holidays and health plans, and just plain recognition of your integral role in the life of the hospital.

Hospital clerical workers care about people--that's why they work in hospitals. Isn't it time you cared about yourself just a little. Start caring today -- check out what SEIU, the nation's largest union of hospital workers, can do for you. Mail the attached card today and get started toward a better deal for yourself right away.

AUTHORIZATION FOR REPRESENTATION

LOCAL 47, SERVICE EMPLOYEES INTERNATIONAL UNION, AFL-CIO

I hereby authorize Local 47, Service Employees International Union, AFL-CIO, to represent me for the purpose of collective bargaining with my employer, and to negotiate and conclude all agreements respecting wages, hours and other terms and conditions of employment. I understand that this card can be used by the Union to obtain recognition from my employer without an election.

NAME _____ DATE _____

EMPLOYEED AT _____

JOB TITLE _____DEPT. OR DIV. _____

DATE HIRED _____ HOURS PER WEEK _____ HOURLY WAGE RATE _____ SHIFT _____

HOME ADDRESS _____CITY OR TOWN _____ ZIP _____

SIGNATURE _____ PHONE _____

READ BEFORE SIGNING

LOOK WHAT'S HAPPENING TO YOUR HOSPITAL...

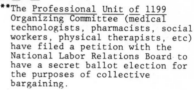

**The <u>Professional Unit of 1199</u> Organizing Committee (medical technologists, pharmacists, social workers, physical therapists, etc) have filed a petition with the National Labor Relations Board to have a secret ballot election for the purposes of collective bargaining.

**The <u>Technical Unit of 1199</u> (LPN's, technicians, etc.) are revising a petition to be filed with the N.L.R.B. for the same purpose.

**Since Nov. 19, 1973, the engineering and maintenance employees of Newport Hospital have enjoyed all the benefits of 1199 membership -- comprehensive medical benefits, significant pay increases, democratic grievance procedure, and full seniority & pension rights.
****

JOIN LOCAL 1199 TODAY!

Don't Be Left Out In The Cold!

Technical, professional and maintenance employees all know the value of organization. They know that behind the door meetings with Mr. Healy will not guarantee their hard earned right to job security and better working conditions. They know that only an organization run by and for hospital employees like 1199 can defend and preserve these rights.

Now the Newport Hospital administration makes all the decisions while YOU do all the work. As members of 1199, employees and administrators sit down as equals to negotiate the <u>employees</u> working conditions. During negotiations, decisions are made after BOTH sides have had their voices heard.

Now, only one side has the final work.

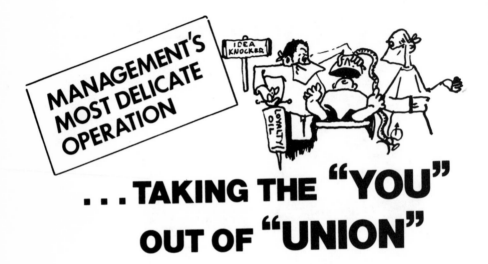

If management of Arlington Memorial Hospital has their way, YOU and
YOUR fellow employees will NEVER receive the benefits of a
GUARANTEED UNION CONTRACT.

Regardless of what Management says, REMEMBER, its YOU and YOUR
families wages and working conditions, as outlined below, that
will be IMPROVED through a UNION CONTRACT!

     .....LIVING WAGES   .....FULL PAID HOLIDAYS

     .....EMPLOYER PAID INSURANCE .....PENSION PROGRAM

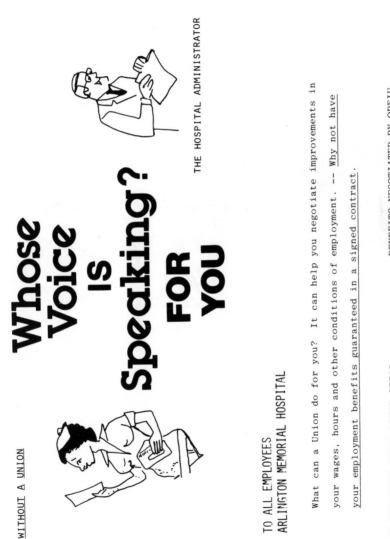

WITHOUT A UNION

THE HOSPITAL ADMINISTRATOR

Whose Voice is Speaking? FOR YOU

TO ALL EMPLOYEES
ARLINGTON MEMORIAL HOSPITAL

What can a Union do for you? It can help you negotiate improvements in your wages, hours and other conditions of employment. -- Why not have your employment benefits guaranteed in a signed contract.

DO YOU WANT OPEIU LOCAL 277'S BARGAINING PROGRAM FOR YOU?

BENEFITS NEGOTIATED BY OPEIU AT ANOTHER HOSPITAL ARE MUCH HIGHER THAN YOURS:

RUN IT THROUGH
YOUR MIND

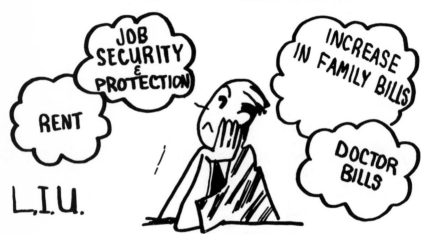

BELOW IS A TEST TO SEE IF YOU NEED
UNION HELP   Please Circle
                                                    One
1.   Do you need a better living wage?   YES   NO

2.   Do you need job security?   YES   NO

3.   Do you need company paid insurance?   YES   NO

4.   Do you need protection from an abusing boss? YES   NO

5.   Do you need cost of living increases in pay? YES   NO

6.   Do you need a system of retirement?   YES   NO

IF YOU'RE IN THE HEALTH CARE FIELD AND YOU HAVE ANSWERED
THE ABOVE QUESTIONS YES-YOU NEED A UNION--AFL-CIO LOCAL 1199

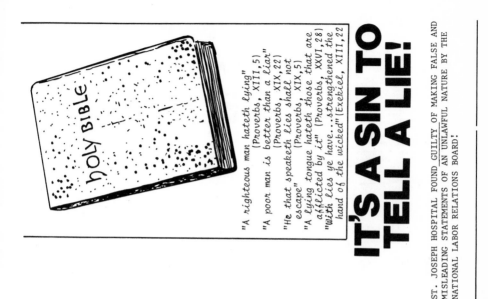

IT'S A SIN TO TELL A LIE!

"A *righteous man hateth lying*"
(*Proverbs, XIII, 5*)
"A *poor man is better than a liar*"
(*Proverbs, XIX, 22*)
"*He that speaketh lies shall not escape*"
(*Proverbs, XIX, 5*)
"*A lying tongue hateth those that are afflicted by it*" (*Proverbs, XXVI, 28*)
"*With lies ye have...strengthened the hand of the wicked*"(*Exekiel, XIII, 22*)

ST. JOSEPH HOSPITAL FOUND GUILTY OF MAKING FALSE AND MISLEADING STATEMENTS OF AN UNLAWFUL NATURE BY THE NATIONAL LABOR RELATIONS BOARD!

ST. JOSEPH'S FOUND GUILTY

On September 19, 1975 the National Labor Relations Board issued a decision in which St. Joseph's Hospital was found guilty of violating your right to a fair election in the following:

LYING

In a letter sent to all employees shortly before the election, and signed by Sister Miriam Regina, the hospital claimed that 1199 contract provided for a single flat rate of pay of $2.40 and $2.50 per hour. This of course is not true and the National Labor Relations Board said that it was clear that the statements made by the Hospital were materially false and misleading and substantially misrepresented the wage rates negotiated and won by the Union in other areas represented.

THREATENING EMPLOYEES

In the weeks before the election, dietary employees were questioned by their supervisor about their views on the union. The N.L.R.B. said such questioning was objectionable. The hospital also had a rule forbidding employees from distributing union literature anywhere on the property and asking employees to tell management if they saw any employee break this rule. The N.L.R.B. said that such a rule was not valid.

1199 believes that the majority of service and maintenance employees at ST. Joseph's want a UNION. We believe that a fair election would prove this. The election held on April 17 was NOT FAIR. BECAUSE OF THE LIES AND THREATS ON THE PART OF THE HOSPITAL, YOUR RIGHTS WERE VIOLATED AND THE FEDERAL GOVERNMENT HAS FOUND THE HOSPITAL GUILTY.

Your right to a fair election will be protected. Things have not at all improved at St. Joseph's without a union as you all know. Stick with 1199 and you will win.

"THE *DOUBLE DEALER UTTERETH LIES*" (*Proverbs, XIV, 25*)

If Newport Hospital Can Do This to Us, When Will YOU BE NEXT??

<u>RESIGNATION</u>: 1 LPN

<u>FIRED</u>: 1 Medical Technologist

<u>RESIGNATION</u>: 6 Nurses, due to overwork and understaffing.

"Forced resignation" is the hospital game to get rid of loyal
employees who buck the Newport Hospital administration and
demand a voice in <u>THEIR</u> hospital. Sometimes the hospital
administrators are <u>not</u> so subtle. Sometimes they out and out
fire a work, like the woman in the lab.

Now Mr. Robert J. Healey, deputy director of Newport Hospital
can freely hire, fire and harass <u>YOU</u>, the unorganized worker.
And because you are not united within an organization that
can and will protect your needs and problems as working people,
the administration can step on you.

What has Healey done since he came to Newport Hospital?

HEALEY PROGRAM FOR NEWPORT HOSPITAL:

Workers are not being replaced when they quit or retire.
Foreced retirement when a worker reached 65 years.
Speed ups on the job.
Forced resignations.
No <u>democratic</u> grievance procedure.
No representation.
Closed door meetings.
Harrassment
****

Want to see an end to The Healey program? Join one of the
1199 Organizing Committees and you'll see some fast improvements.
Workers who have already joined are employees like yourself
who want to put a stop to the Healey way of doing things.

How Can You Join 1199?

If you want to join 1199 National Union of Hospital and Health
Care Workers, or if you just want to get more information about us,
<u>attend a very important meeting</u>:

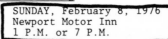
SUNDAY, February 8, 1976
Newport Motor Inn
1 P.M. or 7 P.M.

LPN's and other workers at Women and Infants' Hospital will
talk about their experience with 1199.

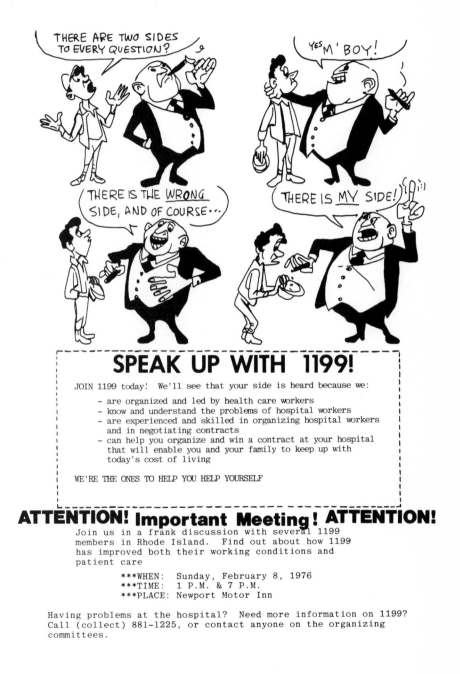

SPEAK UP WITH 1199!

JOIN 1199 today! We'll see that your side is heard because we:

- are organized and led by health care workers
- know and understand the problems of hospital workers
- are experienced and skilled in organizing hospital workers and in negotiating contracts
- can help you organize and win a contract at your hospital that will enable you and your family to keep up with today's cost of living

WE'RE THE ONES TO HELP YOU HELP YOURSELF

ATTENTION! Important Meeting! ATTENTION!

Join us in a frank discussion with several 1199 members in Rhode Island. Find out about how 1199 has improved both their working conditions and patient care

      ***WHEN: Sunday, February 8, 1976
      ***TIME: 1 P.M. & 7 P.M.
      ***PLACE: Newport Motor Inn

Having problems at the hospital? Need more information on 1199? Call (collect) 881-1225, or contact anyone on the organizing committees.

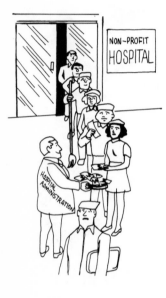

Yes, you. You and your fellow hospital employees contribute millions of dollars each year to the support of the nation's hospitals. How?

Through your low wages. Long hours. Poor working conditions.

Through your lack of a decent health care plan.

Through the lack of a decent retirement plan.

You (like all hospital employees) help to provide a vital service to the American people. You share in maintaining an important and necessary function in the life of every community in the nation.

Yet all the statistics show that you are among the lowest paid workers in your community--when you aren't actually the lowest.

Recent figures show that unorganized hospital workers lag 60 cents an hour (often more) behind the average American worker. When you multiply that by the number of hospital workers it mounts into the millions.

In effect, your low wages and poor working conditions are a forced contribution. Its a subisdy from those who can lease afford it for the benefit of those who can afford it far easier.

You can end this forced charity--as hundreds of thousands of hospital workers have--by joining SEIU. If you're interested in learning more about SEIU and what it can do for you, mail the attached card.

---------------(TEAR OFF AT DOTTED LINE AND MAIL. NO STAMP NECESSARY.)------------------

HOSPITAL WORKERS ORGANIZING COMMITTEE

SERVICE EMPLOYEES INTERNATIONAL UNION, AFL-CIO

YES, I'd like to know more about how SEIU can help me get higher wages and better benefits.

___ Please send me more information.

___ I will help form an SEIU Committee. Please have a union representative contact me.

My name is: ....

My address is: ....Zip...........Phone..........

I work at: ....

Address: ....

SIGNED: ....

AUTHORIZATION FOR REPRESENTATION

LOCAL 47, SERVICE EMPLOYEES INTERNATIONAL UNION, AFL-CIO

I hereby authorize Local 47, Service Employees International Union, AFL-CIO to represent me for the purpose of collective bargaining with my employer and to negotiate and conclude all agreements respecting wages, hours and other terms and conditions of employment. I understand that this card can be used by the Union to obtain recognition from my employer without an election.

NAME	DATE
EMPLOYED AT	
JOB TITLE	DEPT. OR DIV,
DATE HIRED	HOURS PER WEEK HOURLY WAGE RATE SHIFT
HOME ADDRESS	CITY OR TOWN ZIP
SIGNATURE	PHONE

TEAR OFF AT DOTTED LINE AND MAIL. NO STAMP NECESSARY

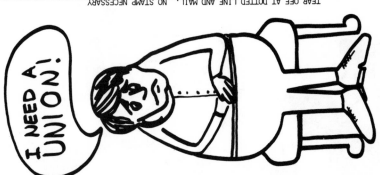

ARE YOU MAKING ENOUGH MONEY?

ENOUGH TO FEED YOUR FAMILY THE WAY YOU'D LIKE TO? ENOUGH TO TAKE CARE OF ALL YOUR BILLS? ENOUGH TO LIVE WHERE YOU'D LIKE TO?

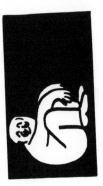

THE ODDS ARE YOU'RE NOT. HOSPITAL PAY HAS ALWAYS BEEN BAD, AND TODAY INFLATION MAKES A BAD SITUATION WORSE.

THERE'S A WAY TO GET A BIGGER PAY-CHECK—AND BETTER BENEFITS AND TREATMENT ON THE JOB, TOO. IT'S CALLED SERVICE EMPLOYEES INTERNATIONAL UNION, AFL-CIO—THE NATION'S LARGEST UNION OF HEALTH CARE WORKERS.

THE ODDS ARE THAT SEIU'S HALF-MILLION MEMBERS IN THE UNITED STATES AND CANADA ARE LIVING BETTER LIVES THAT YOU ARE. WHY? BECAUSE WHILE THEY HAVE UNION CONTRACTS THAT GUARANTEE REGULAR WAGE INCREASES, YOU DON'T.

IF YOU WANT A CHANCE TO WIN BETTER WAGES AND BENEFITS FOR YOURSELF AND YOUR CO-WORKERS, VOTE FOR THE AFL-CIO'S SEIU—THE LARGEST UNION OF HEALTH CARE EMPLOYEES IN THE NATION. UNLESS, OF COURSE, YOU DON'T THINK YOU NEED THE MONEY.

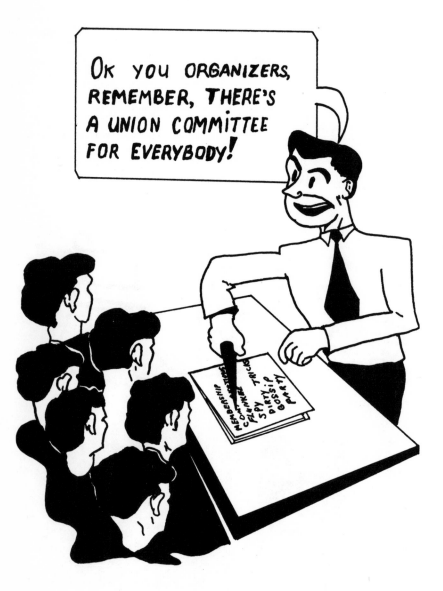

Chapter 6

PARDON ME, BUT YOUR SLIP IS SHOWING
or
PITFALLS TO AVOID

Sitting alone in his/her office the supervisor/administrator is reflecting on the recent day's events:

> Damn, why did I even open my mail today! Got this blasted union petition! Never thought they would get enough cards to do this. We have worked hard to stop this thing—now my labor lawyer tells me that I have gotta hold a meeting with all my supervisors. What in hell am I gonna tell 'em—in fact what am I gonna tell them to tell their people?

Such is the dilemma facing all supervisors in successful union organizing drives. The union already has achieved a major victory by winning the first round. They obtained enough employee signatures on union authorization cards to force a union election. As a result of this defeat, the hospital will now enter into the most difficult part of the campaign. Untold hours must go into the war against the union, and one of the most important understandings a supervisor must have is what he/she can and cannot do. This chapter will seek to give a few guidelines in that direction.

WHAT A SUPERVISOR CAN SAY AND DO

The federal labor law specifically *guarantees the supervisor the right of free speech* during union organizing drives. Too much has been written about the negative, what the supervisor should not do. The end result is that supervisors are often so scared by lawyers and consultants and so afraid of an unfair labor practice that they do nothing. The truth is there is more that can be done than cannot. Section (8)(c) NLRA reads,

> The expressing of any views, argument, or opinion, or the dissemination thereof, whether in written, printed, graphic, or visual form, shall not constitute or be evidence of an unfair labor practice under any of the provisions of this Act, if such expression contains no threat of reprisal or force or promise of benefits.

You can tell your employees that if a majority of them select an outside organization (the union), the hospital will have to deal with it concerning all their problems involving wages, hours, and other conditions of employment. You may advise them that you would prefer to continue dealing with them directly instead of going through a middleman. Also, you may state definitely your opposition to unionization and request that your employees vote against the union. You can criticize a union and state *facts* concerning it. The following, an excerpt from an address given at a hospital where the Teamsters were attempting to organize, is an example of what is permitted.

> ...and this so-called hospital union composed of the truckers has historically been loaded with graft and deceit. For example in November of 1975 teams of investigators from the Labor Department and the FBI and the Internal Revenue Service were engaged in a massive nationwide investigation of the union's financial dealings, particularly with the underworld. That's just another episode in the Teamsters dealings which ran afoul of the law. Look at some of the crooked union leaders. David Beck, one time president of the Teamsters, went to jail for misuse of what would be your pension funds; his successor, Hoffa, went to jail for jury tampering, and now his successor, Fitzsimmons, is under investigation for pouring nearly $60 million dollars of pension funds into Rancho La Costa, a plush 5,600-acre country club and resort near San Diego, operated, in part, by former bootlegger and

gambler Morris Dalitz and Allard Roen, who is an admitted stock swindler.

And where do your monies go that you pay into the union each month? . . .To people like Frank Fitzsimmons, who owns a palatial home worth at least $250,000. . .to other shaky crime-controlled deals, to people like Jimmy Hoffa, if they could ever find Jimmy Hoffa. I ask you, is this the type of organization you want to represent your interests and those of your families?

That speech was pretty strong, but it was legal and *well* received.

You can tell employees that if anybody causes them any trouble on the job or tries to pressure or threaten them into signing a union card, for them to let you know; you will see that it is stopped. Tell the employees that the federal government will punish any union that tries to restrain or coerce employees in their right not to join the union.

You can tell the employees they just cannot "try the union out to see if they like it." Once the union is in, it is almost impossible to get rid of it.

Tell employees you and others at the hospital are always willing to talk about any problem that the employee has or about any subject that is of interest to them. With a union they would have to take their personal problems to a union steward first.

Discuss with the employees the wages, benefits, and working conditions presently given, and how they compare with others in the area. You do not have to let the union get off with showing their "pet" contract from some area remote from your organization. It is good to point out the benefits, wages, etc. now received by the employee are without payment of any union dues or fees to the union. Let the employee know the hospital is not required to continue its present benefits if a union is successful in an election. Whatever benefits the employees receive after the union is successful must be negotiated with the union. The benefits employees receive after the union is successful could be less, more, or the same as the present. No law requires the hospital to continue its present benefits in any contract negotiated with the union. If the union's campaign propaganda to employees contains a promise of obtaining increased wages and if the hospital believes that such wages would seriously impair the successful operation of the hospital, that view should be made clear to the employees.

Tell employees about any untrue or misleading statements made by the union in handbills or any other media. You can correct any false statements made by unions. You can always give your employees the truth, and you can pass out or otherwise distribute any articles written about unions (preferably those about the union in question). Always include the date and source of such information.

Tell employees that merely signing a union authorization card or application for membership does not mean that they must support or vote for a union in an election. Remind employees that anyone who considers joining the union will not get any special treatment or special favors of any type over those who do not sign or belong.

Tell employees that the union cannot guarantee them anything. A union can just promise benefits; only management can deliver them. Tell employees that neither union nor law requires your hospital to agree to any demand it does not want to meet.

Spell out the disadvantages of belonging to a union, such as the loss of income due to strikes (give an accurate account of strikes at other facilities if possible) and the requirements to serve on a picket line. There are also personal expenses to be considered as part of membership, such as the high cost of union dues and union fines, some possible union assessments, or special initiation fees.

You can tell employees federal law permits your hospital to hire permanent replacements for anyone who goes out on an economic strike called by the union, and that where there are unions, there are usually strikes. Remind them that they will not be able to draw any wages from the hospital if they are out on strike. Tell them the union can fine its members for crossing the picket line, even though the employee does not want to strike.

You can discuss seniority provisions of union contracts, which can handicap ambitious or highly skilled employees from advancing to higher positions according to their own abilities. A strong argument is that there is nothing a union can do for an employee that the employee cannot do for himself, cheaper and more directly. Tell employees unions cannot guarantee job security; job security is guaranteed by an employee's efforts at the job he/she was hired to do.

You should tell employees that the union has a legal right to go into court and sue its membership to collect fines levied by the union on the employee for violation of various union rules, such as crossing union picket lines. You can tell the employees that unionized members are always subject to and frequently are taxed with increased union assessments, in addition to periodic dues. Often persons working in unionized organizations find they must provide money for employees in other organizations who are out on strike.

You can tell employees unions are against employee overtime, just as a matter of principle. Unions prefer to have more dues-paying members working regular hours, as against fewer members working overtime.

Employees should be told your opinions about unions and union activities. You can do this in unflattering language. You can (factually) tell employees about any personal experiences you have had with unions, especially the union seeking to represent the employees. If appropriate, you can tell the employees that you feel the international union will try to take over the local union or, at a minimum, try to influence its local members.

Tell employees anything you know about the union or its officers, even of a critical nature such as jury tampering, theft of employee pension funds, and the extremely high salaries for union officers. You can tell employees what you think of a union position on any issue, whether it is fair or unfair. Remember to mention what you think of the union organizers and whether you feel they are doing the right thing.

You can point out that a union is anything but a democracy. It is a highly political institution. Those in the hospital who are helping to organize the union will invariably end up becoming the union favorites and the stewards. In other words, these people have definite self-serving interests and personal gain possibilities from hospital unionization. Tell employees they do not have to sign any unionization authorization cards that are passed out or mailed to their homes. Make an analogy between signing the card and signing a blank check—you can never tell what it is going to cost. Stress to employees that they do not have to talk to union organizers at work or at their homes unless they want to.

You can tell employees why the hospital is doing something which may be under attack by the union. Campaign strongly and sincerely against the union in the hospital's campaign. Remember, you can talk to employees in groups on hospital property and on hospital time, so long as the discussion is not made within the twenty-four silence period preceding the election. You can distribute printed counterunion material to employees at work or send it to their homes, even though they might receive it within the twenty-four-hour period.

An important tactic is demanding that the union organizers restrict their efforts to secure employee-members outside the health care facility's grounds. (Of course, an employee can discuss the union on nonworking time and try to persuade coworkers to join, even if he/she is on the hospital's property, as long as such activity does not interfere with his/her job.) You can enforce a rule restricting the distribution of all literature (union and nonunion) to the nonworking areas of the hospital, and you can enforce any rules requiring that the oral solicitation of membership be conducted outside working time. Remember, too, that you can enforce all the hospital's rules and regulations in accordance with customary past practices, regardless of whether an employee is a union or nonunion member. You can layoff, discipline, and discharge for cause, as long as such action follows customary practice and is done without regard to union or nonunion membership. Assignments of overtime, shift preference, or preferred work can be made if done without reference to the employee's participation or nonparticipation in union activities.

You can tell employees about the NLRB election procedures and the importance of every vote. If only a few vote and they are for the union, the union could win the election, even though the majority did not favor its representation. Tell the employees their vote is secret and that there is absolutely means of finding out how they voted. While stressing these facts, you can tell the employees that you and the hospital are seeking a "no" vote in the election and that you neither want nor need a union. You can point out that if a union should get into your facility, it would not work to the employees' best interest; in fact, it could work to their disadvantage.

Finally, you can tell employees that you will oppose the union by each and every legal and proper means at your disposal—that you will fight any attempt to break up the good working relationships that exist in your health care facility.

WHAT FEW THINGS SUPERVISORS CANNOT DO

Obviously there are a great number of things a hospital supervisor can do in the war against unions. We would be remiss, though, if we neglected the few things the supervisor cannot do.

You cannot promise a pay increase, promotion, betterment, benefit, or special favor if the employees stay out of the union or vote against it.

You cannot threaten an employee in any way, directly or indirectly by (1) saying the hospital will be closed if the union comes in; (2) saying employees will be fired, laid off, or given a less favorable job; or (3) discriminating against an employee because of his/her union activities.

You cannot interrogate employees (never call them into your office alone) concerning their union activities. In particular, do not ask them what they think about a particular representative of the union or unions in general or about others in the work organization engaged in union activities. Also, do not discuss with an employee his direct withdrawal from the union (though you can say why employees should not continue their adherence to the union).

Finally, you cannot stop your employees from wearing their union insignias *unless they are in contact with the public*. Of course, the same rules should apply to antiunion buttons, or similar propaganda.

Now, you know what can and cannot be done. The next thing is to answer an earlier question as to how the union got into the health care organization in the first place, and what it plans to do now that it is there.

Chapter 7

HOW TO CARRY THE BALL
or
STANDING UP TO THE UNION

The recent amendments of the National Labor Relations Act (NLRA) have brought much controversy into the medical world. Suddenly, administrators and line personnel are no longer a health care team but two separate teams, each debating the effect the application of the federal labor laws will have on patient care.

The position being taken by administrators runs parallel to the reasons given in 1944 by the administrators of the Central Dispensary and Emergency Hospital of Washington, D.C.[1] In August 1972, John Painter and Robert Hickey, noted in the health care industry as authorities on labor relations, appeared before the Senate Subcommittee on Labor to testify against H.R. 11356, a bill calling for the inclusion of the health care industry under the Taft-Hartley Act.[2] Painter and Hickey contended that,

> . . .hospitals are not grocery stores, amusement parks, or other enterprises that are regulated by the National Labor Relations Board. They are unique enterprises with unique problems which cannot be compared to those of commercial enterprises. Its services make the nonprofit hospital a valuable member of any community, and the community should not, and indeed cannot, afford to be denied these services. . . . Unlike the profit oriented organizations, the nonprofit hospital's sources of revenue are limited, and it has little or no economic cushion on which to rely. Because of their growing financial strain and the valuable services they provide, nonprofit hospitals should not be subject to the Taft-Hartley provisions.[3]

Furthermore, labor unions will force many institutions to pay wages they cannot afford, and, as a result, some facilities will be forced to close. An increase in wages must result in increased charges to the patient. Also, the hospital is not equipped with countercollective measures found in other enterprises. It cannot, for instance, lock out employees, or cease service.[4]

Hospital strikes, now a reality and not a mere forecast, can have only two possible effects. If the union is successful, the hospital is forced to do what it cannot afford; and this concession has direct effects on patient care. Should the strike be unsuccessful, it succeeds only in interrupting patient care and jeopardizing the lives of patients. It has been said that unions do not win in arbitration, but that hospitals lose.[5]

Looking back at hospital strikes in 1973, it is seen that they have ranged from one to sixty-seven days. In some instances, hospitals were forced to close because of these activities. A strike by nurses at Ingalls Memorial Hospital in Harvey, Illinois, forced the facility to accept only emergency patients. A strike in Britain by 220,000 hospital employees affected no less than 750 hospitals.[6] These instances demonstrate how hospital employees under union control have been willing to strike and close a hospital to benefit themselves.

Unionization of hospital employees will disrupt any concept of a health care team. No one is dispensable in a hospital setting. Administration relies on line personnel to deliver effective health care; employees rely on management to keep the facility an ongoing operation. Unionization will segment the team. Administration will be forced to take a defensive position against employees, while employees will adhere only to their designated tasks. For instance, nurses will not be able to perform a function designated for nurses aides for fear of a grievance filed by an aide. Such has already been the case in union-dominated hospitals.

Another problem with unionization of employees stems from the degree of specialization in a hospital. There are no less than 125 specialized tasks possible in a medical center.[7] If management must deal with unions representing even half this number, it would involve most of the year settling grievances, in arbitration, and attempting to avert strikes. The hospital would be forced to devote a great deal of time to union matters. If the

employees were to organize themselves in a plantwide arrangement, management would spend less time dealing with individual
unions but would still be forced to be prepared for a facilitywide
walkout if one particular group, not necessarily all the employees,
so decided.

Sidney Levine, director of Mount Sinai Hospital of Cleveland
and a member of the joint committee of the American Nurses'
Association and the American Hospital Association aired his concerns before the 10,000 nurses attending the 1975 ANA convention in San Francisco. His comments included:

> The collective bargaining role of the association inevitably
> diminishes the professional role of the association. . . . The
> public will question association credibility when it at-
> tempts to speak for your patients.[8]

Reverend Leo C. Brown, S.J., Ph.D., professor of economics at St.
Louis University, and an arbitrator for labor disputes told the
nurses, "It's one thing when you use the bargaining powers on
issues of economic concerns, another thing on issues of patient
care."[9]

But, the nursing personnel labor leaders definitely had their
own opinions. Last year, the ANA announced its intention to
organize the 800,000 active registered nurses for "professional collective action."[10] Thus, the ANA has accepted its role as a labor
union for the nurses of America.

In answer to the statements by Lewine and Brown, Ada Jacox,
Ph.D., chairperson of the ANA Commission on Economic and
General Welfare of the ANA replied:

> This tactic of labeling certain behaviors as "unprofes-
> sional" has been so widely used in the past to control
> nurses. How much respect have hospital administrators
> had generally for us as a profession. . . . It is a self-serving
> device for hospital administrators to tell nurses or any
> other professionals that their image as professionals will
> be tarnished if they challenge the authority of the ad-
> ministrators. . . . We will decide for ourselves how best to
> express our professionalism.[11]

PROMISES MADE BY UNIONS

Unions and union organizers tend to argue for unionizing by stating certain promises that seek to capitalize on present management weaknesses. Beginning with the most common promises and appeals made to your employees, unions usually promise that:

1. The union will see that management policies are uniformly applied and that fair and just treatment will be afforded to all employees.
2. The union will make management "shape up." They will do this by requiring good management practices, such as grievance procedures, which management should be doing now but is not.
3. There will be better communication all the way around. No longer will the employees feel they are out in the cold. The union can bargain directly at the top, so workers will be more aware of management policies and possible changes.
4. The unions will serve as agents for promoting policy changes desired by employees. They will not allow management to maintain the status quo.
5. A fair grievance procedure will be established by the union, which will allow an employee an impartial "court of appeals." The union will serve as the advocate for the employee who has been the object of discrimination.
6. Promotion and transfer policies will be fairly established; no longer will the supervisor's "fair-haired boy" be the one promoted. The union will stop "favoritism."
7. The union will foster greater employee personal development. It will see that job enlargement, self-actualization, creativity, etc. are made the direct concern of management.
8. Improved and more equitable wages will be insured by union representation.
9. Improved benefits for all employees will be installed in the health care facility's compensation program.

10. The seniority rights of the long service employee will be protected. The union will insure that the more senior employees will get preferential treatment.

11. Job security will be attained so an employee cannot be fired simply because of some supervisor's whim or fancy.

12. Working conditions, hours, equipment, environment, etc. will be improved. Scheduling of work time will be supervised by the union to insure equitable treatment.

13. The employees will be given involvement in the operation of the health care facility. They will (through the union) be a part of determining the standards of care for the institution as well as helping to run other day to day operations.

14. As a result of having a "piece of the action" and a determining hand in the decision-making process, the authoritarian rule of the administration will be overthrown, and democracy will be the result.

15. The substantial achievements in all the items above will strengthen employee morale and worker unity.

It would seem that if management understood the union "points" above there would truly be no "need for a union." Unfortunately, too many managers/supervisors make the fatal mistake at looking at the employee through their own "management-colored" glasses. A recent study by the authors of twenty-five health care facilities in the greater Dallas, Texas, area demonstrated that supervision is seldom in touch with the workers' needs and desires. One hundred supervisors (nurses, administrators, physicians) were asked to rank the importance of a number of job factors (pay, meaningful work, being "in on things," etc.) as they felt their employees would rank them. Supervision unanimously selected pay as number one, meaningful work as number two, and "being in on things" as number fourteen (there were fifteen items). When four hundred employees were asked to rank their own preferences, they placed as number one "being in on things." Other supervision/nonsupervision rankings were equally mismatched.

If management continually conceives of the employee's perspective from an entirely different point of view, management can count on union activity. Supervisors should not make the mistake of assuming that if they hear no complaints there are none. Management should know and be aware as much as possible of those things that the employees feel are important. To do this management must reduce the "management gap" through communication, an important area discussed in Chapter 9.

FACING THE PROBLEMS OF UNION LITERATURE AND AUTHORIZATION CARDS

Many hospitals and supervisors linger in the belief that it is best to do nothing and say nothing about the union until they are forced to do so. The theory is that if the hospital and its supervisors keep its union resistance low-keyed, then the employees will not get involved themselves.

At best, this seems an exercise in wishful thinking; and at worst it is a dangerous approach. If the goal of the hospital and its supervisors is to remain nonunion, then certain preventive measures must be implemented before the union organizational drive begins. In addition, the first major battle to be waged when the union shows up is to educate employees about the serious consequences that can result from signing union authorization cards.

The battle is a two-stage, perhaps a three-stage, proposition. First, the hospital must implement preventive measures. Second, the hospital must convince its employees not to sign union authorization cards; and failing that, the hospital and every supervisor must wage an effective campaign to win the NLRB-supervised election.

To do any of these necessary steps effectively, the hospital must enlist and rely on every supervisor employed. Therefore, as a supervisor on the front line with the employees on a day to day basis, you are in the best position to ascertain the early signs of union activity among your own employees.

The following list of problems are those that you may be faced with any day now; and, therefore, you are provided suggested approaches for successfully dealing with each specific problem.

Problem: Union literature appears on hospital union bulletin boards.

Solution: Calmly remove the union materials from the bulletin boards, and immediately notify the personnel director or administrator. Avoid making a search or inquiry as to the identity of who posted the union materials on the bulletin boards.

Problem: A person is distributing union handbills or is soliciting members for the union.

Solution: If a union organizer is engaging in union activities on the property of the hospital, ask him to leave the premises immediately. If he does not, immediately contact the personnel director or administrator. Confiscate any union materials left on the hospital's property, but allow the union organizer to take it with him if he wishes. If you witness an employee handing out union handbills or soliciting members for the union, immediately report such conduct to the personnel director or administrator. If the employee is engaging in such activity on his working time or during the working time of those with whom he is in contact, he should be told to stop such activities, and that he is subject to certain disciplinary action for using hospital time in such a manner.

Problem: An employee publically indicates prounion sentiments to you.

Solution: Report such comments or discussions immediately to the personnel director or administrator. Do not argue with the employee, but firmly state your opposition to the union concept.

Problem: An employee comes to you and says that he is acting as a representative of a group of employees.

Solution: Listen to the employee's statement covering the complaint. Thank him/her for bringing it up, and tell the employee you will get back to him/her shortly. Remind the employee of the availability of supervisors for the discussion of any grievance, and the grievance procedure. But report the employee complaint promptly to the personnel director or administrator for action and resolution.

Problem: An employee reports to you that he has been invited to a union meeting off the hospital premises.

Solution: Listen to the employee's report but do not ask questions or interrogate the employee; especially do not discourage the employee from attending. Nor should you show any annoyance. Report the incident to the personnel director or administrator as soon as possible.

Some hospitals face the issue of the union authorization card head on by providing all employees with the following list of questions and answers about union authorization cards:

Question: The union man asked me to sign a card. What does the card mean?

Answer: The card is called an authorization card. It is a legal statement that says you want the union to represent you. Be sure you have all the facts before you sign one. It is a very serious matter.

Question: What does the union do with those cards they are asking us to sign?

Answer: They use them two ways—both are SERIOUS AND LEGAL MATTERS. They might use them to ask the federal government to hold an election, or they might use them to try to force the hospital to recognize them. Do not sign anything until you are sure you know all the facts in this matter.

Question: Why is the union trying to get us to sign those cards?

Answer: They are trying to SELL you something that is going to cost you money (dues, fees, assessments, and fines). Be very careful about any promises they are making. Be sure to get all the facts before you sign anything.

Question: The union said that the card is only to get more information. Is that true?

Answer: Absolutely not. The card might be used for serious legal matters. Be sure you get all the facts before you sign anything.

Question: The union said I have to sign a card to vote. Is that true?

Answer: Absolutely not. If there is an election in your group, you will get to vote whether you signed a card or not. Do not put your name on anything before you get all the facts.

Question: The union said the cards will only be used to force an election. Is that true?

Answer: Not necessarily. The cards might be used to try to force the hospital to recognize the union without an election. Signing a card is a serious and legal matter. Be sure you have all the facts.

Question: The union said if I do not sign now, I will not have a job if they get in. Is that true?

Answer: Absolutely not. Your job will always depend only on your performance, union or not. Inform me should the union tell you this again. Report this to the personnel director and administrator.

Question: Can I ever be forced into signing a card?

Answer: No. You have a legal right not to sign the card.

Question: What if I get pressured or threatened about signing a card?

Answer: Please let your supervisor know immediately. The hospital guarantees you 100 percent protection of your legal rights.

Question: I signed one of those cards, and now I want it back. What should I do?

Answer: I am not sure. If I were you, I would contact the National Labor Relations Board for advice.

In addition, the hospital can mail to each employee's home a letter outlining the position of the hospital. An example follows:

> We do not want a union, and we do not need a union at our hospital. It is our firm intention to oppose this union, and to prevent it from coming in here, by every proper and legal means.

> This union matter is of grave concern to our hospital. It should also be a matter of serious concern to you and your family, because it is our deepest belief that if the union is

successful in our hospital, it would not work to the community's benefit, the hospital's benefit, or to your benefit.

We want to make it clear that it is not necessary now and it will not be necessary for any employee to belong to the union to work in our hospital. If any employee does show an interest in joining a union, he/she is not going to get any advantages or any preferred treatment of any type over those employees who do not join or belong to the union.

If the union causes any employee any trouble by intimidating or coercing the employee in his/her right to refrain from belonging to the union (such as telling the employee he/she will be without a job for not joining), we will take all legal actions to stop this unfair labor practice on the part of the union immediately. Please report any such action immediately.

We have always respected the rights, privileges, and the individual dignity of all our employees. We shall continue to do so regardless of the future activities of this or any other union.

NOTES

1. Vernon Coleman, "Can Anyone Be A Health Professional and A Trade Unionist?" *Nursing Mirror,* Vol. 54, No. 1 (August 30, 1974): 41.
2. Dennis Dale Pointer, "Hospital Labor Relations Legislation: An Examination and Critique of Public Policy," *Hospital Progress,* Vol. 54, No. 1 (January 1973): 71-75.
3. John Pointer and Robert J. Hickey, "Arguments Against NLRB Regulation of Hospitals," *Hospital Progress,* Vol. 54, No. 7 (July 1973): 47-53.
4. *Ibid.*
5. *Ibid.*
6. Owen Parker, Assistant Administrator, St. Mary's Hospital, personal interview (July 22, 1975).
7. John Pointer and Robert J. Hickey, "Arguments Against NLRB Regulation of Hospitals," *op. cit.*
8. D. F. Phillips, "Taft-Hartley: What to Expect," *Hospitals,* Vol. 48, No. 13 (July 1, 1974): 18a-18d.

9. "The A.N.A.—Can A Professional Association Be A Trade Union, Too?" *Hospitals,* Vol. 48, No. 17 (September 1974): 103-115.

10. *Ibid.*

11. *Ibid.*

Sample Union
Flyers and Handbills

1199 NATIONAL UNION OF HOSPITAL AND HEALTH CARE EMPLOYEE MEMBERS WHO WORK AT WOMEN AND INFANTS' HOSPITAL, FALMOUTH NURSING HOME, THE JEWISH HOME, COUNTRY GARDENS NURSING HOME, ADAMS DRUG, PARKVIEW NURSING HOME, NEWPORT HOSPITAL (MAINTENANCE) AND THE NEWLY ORGANIZED BANNISTER HOUSE   HAVE WON:

*Free & Complete Health Benefits
-Hospital, Surgical & Medical Coverage
-Payments for out-patient services
-Disability Pay of 2/3's weekly pay up to 26 weeks if employee is unable to work.
-Life insurance covering one year's pay; a maximum of $12,000.
-Free prescription drugs.
-Payment for eye-glasses and dental care.
-Decent retirement benefits.
-Uniform allowance.
-Improved Vacations and sick leave.
-Premium pay for holidays.
-Automatic Cost-of-living increases.

GRIEVANCE PROCEDURE
To provide Job Security, Real Rights for all employees. The right to have representation and to appeal any unfair management action to an Impartial Arbitrator.

Seniority Rights
Full seniority rights for all employees; seniority to begin from original date of hire. No discrimination in granting job promotions, weekends off, etc.
*Job Training and Promotions.
*Pay increases of $24 to $40 a week.

THESE BENEFITS CAN BE YOURS--JUST FOLLOW THE LESSON LEARNED BELOW:

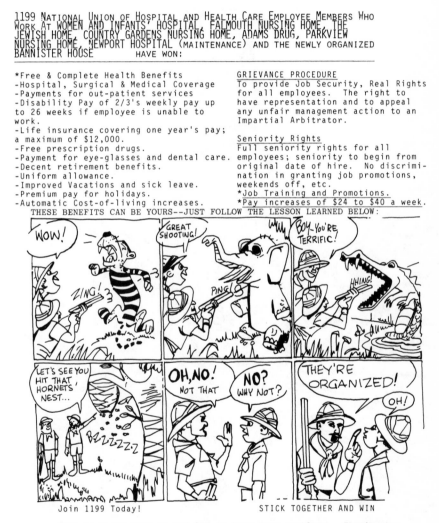

Join 1199 Today!   STICK TOGETHER AND WIN

Keep in touch with us and let us hear your problems. That's what we are here for. Call collect anytime (861-1225) 1199 National Union of Hospital and Health Care Employees, 212 Union St., Providence Rhode Island.

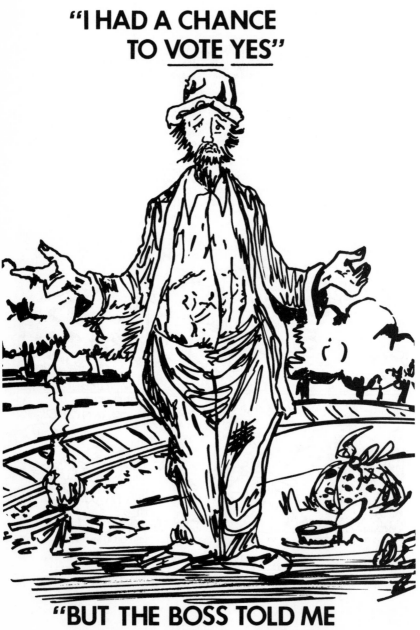

Hospital Administrators, Doctors, Religious Authorities, Newspaper Editors.

Here's what some important people who aren't unionists say about unions for hospital workers —

Hospital Unions Are Good

"Unions in hospitals are a good thing. Where conditions once were dreadful, unions have improved them which in turn makes it possible to attract a higher grade of employee...."

Hon. Charles Daley, former Minister of Labor for Ontario, Canada in "Saturday Night."

Unions Help Attract Stable Worker Force

"The caliber of the workers has improved since the union came in. The union gave security and we got more stable people. Before unionization, we got last-chance people, men and women who couldn't find another job."

Ray Amberg, director, University of Minnesota hospital, Minneapolis, and president of the American Hospital Association, quoted in "Wall Street Journal."

More Benefits Tomorrow

"In 1962 the average hospital worker was making... about 43 percent less than his fellow industrial worker. Hospital unions are fighting today for recognition; tomorrow they may be fighting—and striking—for better pay, a shorter work week, and more fringe benefits."

Ray E. Brown, vice president, University of Chicago; past president, American Hospital Association.

"Isn't it Unfair and Inhuman?"

"Isn't it unfair and inhuman to ask hospital workers to help meet hospital deficits by accepting substandard wages?"

New York "Herald Tribune," as quoted in "Modern Hospital."

Should Workers Be Philanthropists?

"But why should workers performing the same kind of jobs as in private employment be asked to be philanthropists by accepting much lower wages and the human suffering that follows? And why should collective bargaining be denied them when that is a policy overwhelmingly approved

by the American public?

Those wise in the ways of labor-management relations know that, given widespread employee dissatisfaction and a truly representative organization, it is far better to deal with a union than to resist it. Formal grievance procedures and two-way communication alone can often do a great deal to increase morale and effective job performance. To slam the door shut on such advantages may well have precisely the opposite effect in the voluntary hospitals."

New York "Times" editorial, taken from "Public Health Economics."

For Equity and Fair Play

"In large scale hospital operations, some equivalent of collective bargaining or organized employee representative spokesmanship with real powers is essential to equity, fair play, and effective two-way communication...."

Ordway Tread, vice-president of Harper & Brothers, N.Y., quoted in "Modern Hospital."

Hospital Employees Are Entitled

"At the very least, hospital employees are entitled to negotiate an agreement with their employers preferably through a bona fide union of their own choice. They also have a right to ask that this agreement be put in writing, so that there will be no reasonable doubt as to its meaning and scope...."

Msgr. George G. Higgins, in "The Catholic Standard."

"Wage Scales Are Low"

"If we are going to have hospital labor-management peace in the decade ahead, both sides are going to have to face some hard realities. First, hospital wage scales on the whole are low... When it comes time to consider how best to use the precious dollars you have under your control, I urge you to... give a high priority to the legitimate needs of (your) employees so that they, in turn, will have the desire to give their very best to the hospital...."

W.J. Usery, Jr., Director, Federal Mediation and Conciliation Service, in a speech to the American Health Congress.

(Tear off at dotted line and mail. No stamp necessary.)

- -

AUTHORIZATION FOR REPRESENTATION
Local 47, Service Employees International Union, AFL-CIO

I hereby authorize Local 47, Service Employees International Union, AFL-CIO, to represent me for the purpose of collective bargaining with my employer, and to negotiate and conclude all agreements respecting wages, hours and other terms and conditions of employment. I understand that this card can be used by the Union to obtain recognition from my employer without an election.

Name _____ Date _____
(Please Print)

Employed at _____

Job Title _____ Dept. or Div. _____

Date Hired _____ Hours per week _____ Hourly Wage Rate _____ Shift ☐ Day ☐ Evening ☐ Night

Home address _____ City or town _____ Zip _____

Signature _____ Phone _____
(Sign Do Not Print)   READ BEFORE SIGNING

Sample Management
Information

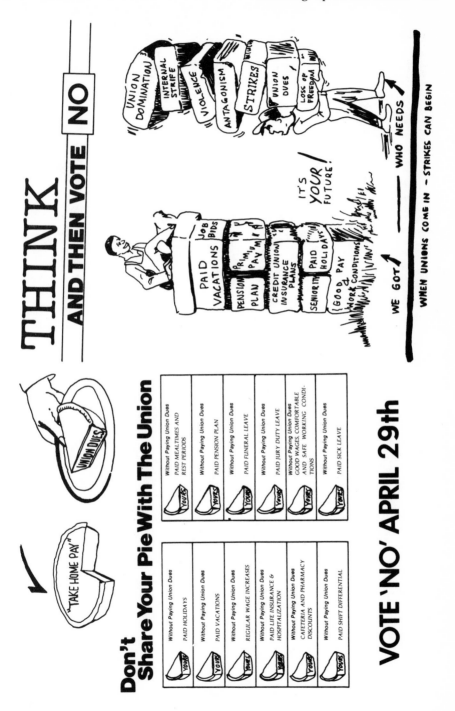

Chapter 8

THE LONGEST DAY

It is only 2:00 p.m., and the employees have been voting since 8:00 a.m. this morning. It already has been a long day, but after only a few more hours you will know the result. The hospital's labor lawyer told you that the vote counting is open to the public after the polls close at 4:00 p.m. today. The National Labor Relations Board (NLRB) agent conducting the election will count all the ballots on the spot, and the hospital will have won or lost the election.

It does not seem right, you think, that the union only needs a majority of the votes cast to win. You would feel better if it took a majority of all eligible votes. Every supervisor in the hospital has been involved in this union debate, some more than others. You have all put in a lot of time and effort to present the hospital's side of the union question to the employeee. You have personally talked to all the employees in your department. Now there is nothing left to do but wait and hope.

A labor union trying to organize your hospital! That really shocked all of you. Of course, you had read about the unionization of hospitals, and there had been television news programs about its various activities. The union's lawyers said the largest, richest and most aggressive labor union in the country was trying to organize hospitals in your area. It has already filed petitions with the NLRB for two other hospitals in the city; you will be number three. Other hospitals will be involved shortly, but right now it is your hospital. You know you must fight to prevent the union from winning the election at your hospital.

You all had many questions for the union's lawyer, and he gave you a long written list of "do's" and "don'ts" to study. He refused,

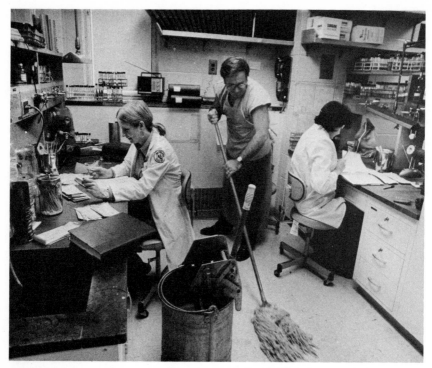

New York Daily News. Reprinted with permission.

Dr. Henry Isenberg mops floor in nurses' station at Long Island Jewish Hospital yesterday.

however, to discuss contract negotiations or possible changes if the union won, instead telling you only to work on winning the election if you could. From that day on the only thing in your minds was a mark in the "no" column on the ballot.

All those preparations occurred only two months ago, but it seems more like two years ago. All the long hours and hard work, and the outside management consultants, are past; soon the election will be over.

It is 4:05 p.m. in the hospital cafeteria; and it looks as if every supervisor in the hospital is here, along with many employees as well. The representative from the local NLRB regional office introduces himself and says that he has been present all day during the balloting, which officially has closed. He breaks open the cardboard ballot box, opens each ballot, and places it face down in front of him. After that, he takes each one and reads it aloud, "yes" or "no," then puts it in a stack for each answer. He counts very slowly. Whenever he gets fifty "yes" or fifty "no" votes, he stops counting and wraps them up in a separate roll. But wait, we soon realize that we have heard more "no's" from the board's agent; we must have won! Soon the counting ends, and the vote totals are announced: 346 for the union, 582 for the hospital. People clap, a few cheer aloud; every supervisor is smiling. A few of the employees look upset and leave the room. The union organizers appear edgy and leave quickly. It is over and you have won. Everyone is excited and talking. It really is over—the union lost the election. It has been a sobering experience, however, because you all realize how easily it could have gone the other way. Just a few more dissatisfied employees, and you could be headed for contract negotiations.

POST ELECTION PROCEDURES

As far as the role of the supervisor is concerned, the union organizing drive is over once the ballots are counted. Hopefully, it is back to patients and business as usual. There will still be problems with some of the employees who supported the union. In every union election that is lost, certain employees will be bad losers and remain malcontent and belligerent.

After the election is over, the supervisor should emphasize that it is now past history and time to think of the future. The supervisor should set the example. Discipline and control should be maintained, but without prejudice or ill-feelings toward a union supporter.

The union has five working days from the date of the election within which to file objections to misconduct by the hospital or the manner in which the election was conducted. If filed, the NLRB regional director assigns someone on his staff to investigate objections to the election. Your hospital labor lawyer will handle any objections the union files.

FINALLY

For you, unionization is out of the picture (at least for the moment), and it is time to get back to your patients and their needs.

Other hospitals, though, might not be so fortunate, and for them it is a whole new era. For your own part it is time to consider a prescription for preventive unionism.

Sample Union
Flyers and Handbills

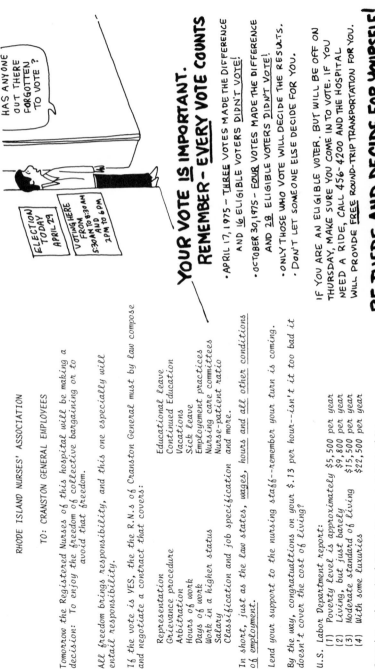

ELECTION TODAY APRIL 29

VOTING HERE FROM 5:30 AM TO 8:30 AM AND 2 PM to 6 PM

HAS ANYONE OUT THERE FORGOTTEN TO VOTE?

RHODE ISLAND NURSES' ASSOCIATION

TO: CRANSTON GENERAL EMPLOYEES

Tomorrow the Registered Nurses of this hospital will be making a decision: To enjoy the freedom of collective bargaining or to avoid that freedom.

All freedom brings responsibility, and this one especially will entail responsibility.

If the vote is YES, the the R.N.s of Cranston General must by law compose and negotiate a contract that covers:

Representation
Grievance procedure
Arbitration
Hours of work
Days of work
Work in a higher status
Salary
Classification and job specification

Educational leave
Continued Education
Vacations
Sick leave
Employement practices
Nursing care committees
Nurse-patient ratio
and more.

In short, just as the law states, wages, hours and all other conditions of employment.

Lend your support to the nursing staff--remember your turn is coming.

By the way, congratualtions on your $.13 per hour--isn't it too bad it doesn't cover the cost of living?

U.S. Labor Department report:
(1) Poverty level is approximately $5,500 per year
(2) Living, but just barely $9,800 per year
(3) Moderate standard of living $15,500 per year
(4) With some luxuries $22,500 per year

Remember, the United States Government says this:
NOW DON'T YOU NEED COLLECTIVE BARGAINING?

P.S. - TO ALL REGISTERED NURSES - VOTE YES FOR COLLECTIVE BARGAINING.

YOUR VOTE IS IMPORTANT.
REMEMBER - EVERY VOTE COUNTS

- APRIL 17, 1975 - THREE VOTES MADE THE DIFFERENCE AND 16 ELIGIBLE VOTERS DIDN'T VOTE!
- OCTOBER 30, 1975 - FOUR VOTES MADE THE DIFFERENCE AND 28 ELIGIBLE VOTERS DIDN'T VOTE!
- ONLY THOSE WHO VOTE WILL DECIDE THE RESULTS.
- DON'T LET SOMEONE ELSE DECIDE FOR YOU.

IF YOU ARE AN ELIGIBLE VOTER, BUT WILL BE OFF ON THURSDAY, MAKE SURE YOU COME IN TO VOTE. IF YOU NEED A RIDE, CALL 456-4200 AND THE HOSPITAL WILL PROVIDE FREE ROUND-TRIP TRANSPORTATION FOR YOU.

BE THERE AND DECIDE FOR YOURSELF!

Section II
PREVENTIVE UNIONIZATION

Chapter 9

HOW TO DESERVE WHAT'S IN STORE FOR YOU
or
BAD MANAGEMENT

Many experts say that no single identifiable cause exists for employees to be receptive to union organizational attempts. It is rather when employees' general feelings about their jobs and working environment are negative that they are responsive to a union's effort. So the real problem is to uncover and consider the employees' subjective perceptions about the hospital. In other words, supervisors too often have an unrealistic sense of their employees' true feelings and actual desires.

All hospitals do not have the same problems that could lead to a union organizing drive. For instance, the discharge of a popular employee in the dietary department of one hospital leads to union organizing activities among all the dietary employees. In other words, the employees themselves may actively seek out the union organizer or make a trip to a local union hall to discuss organizing a particular hospital's employees. Yet in another hospital a layoff or cutback of any employees could result in the remaining employees becoming concerned enough about their job security to seek out a union organizer, or the failure to grant an expected wage increase could cause a union organizing drive.

In other situations, the union organizer just shows up to try and generate employee dissatisfaction and seeks to actively organize a particular hospital's employees. In Houston, Texas, the Teamsters Union made an active citywide solicitation of almost all the hospitals in the area to find the degree of dissatisfaction that existed. They easily gained seven hospital elections by merely getting employees to return mailed authorization cards enclosed in standard brochures.

In other areas of the country, the union can gain major advances in the hospital community by organizing only one major institution in the community. After that successful organizing drive they will spend whatever time necessary to obtain a contract with improved benefits. That contract can then be used as an organizing device for all other hospitals in the community.

Many hospital administrators believe the strongest motivation in all union organizing campaigns is the employees' desire for more wages. However, this simply is not the cause in many, many cases. Over thirty years ago, when the Congress of Industrial Organizations was a very militant organization, they stated, "Workers organize into labor unions not alone for economic motives but also for equally compelling psyschological and social reasons."[1]

MERE SIZE OF HOSPITALS CREATES SPECIAL PROBLEMS

Long ago in the mass production industries, such as automobile production and steel mills, it was discovered that the coldness and impersonality of large plants caused workers to feel alienated from their jobs and not a part of any team. Unions have always thrived on this atmosphere and have used it as the basis for mounting an organizing drive.

The same problem is faced in any large health care institution. The union takes advantage of the situation by pointing to the institution as being large and rich with a low wage scale. Hospitals must be aware that their pay scales rank lower than much of the industrial sector. The unions will certainly use this in their arguments; but even more importantly, they will exploit employee alienation.

The larger institution or hospital is also more likely to have internal fragmentation among various working groups. Employees disassociate themselves from the institution itself or the hospital that employs them and instead, identify with fellow employees in a specialty or subspecialty. In hospitals with fifteen or twenty x-ray technicians, it is natural for these employees to cluster together for socializing as well as working purposes. They are going to develop loyalty to the group rather than to the hospital.

Such fragmentation is often reinforced by the hospital itself, particularly since it has to stress job specialization. Employees respond to these specialization requirements by protecting their specialty and emphasizing its importance over other positions or jobs within the hospital. Thus, a very real danger for hospitals lies among its technical and professional employees. A union will have a special appeal to represent their common interests, which they consider separate from others in the hospital.

THE ANSWER IS COMMUNICATION

There is only one sure answer, and that is communication. Administration and supervisors should talk to their employees on every floor and every shift on a regular basis to find out about their problems and their actual feelings. Supervisors, administrators, and department heads need to be visible to their employees, visible on the floor. They should not wait until the union campaign starts for their subordinates to see them and talk to them for the first time.

Supervisor's Role in the Communication Process

Supervisors in most plants or industrial organizations are clearly designated. But in the hospital community, especially large multipurpose facilities, tthe lines of supervisory authority are often blurred. Registered nurses direct the work of the licensed practical nurses (LPN), aides, and orderlies. On other occasions, the LPNs will direct the work of the aides and orderlies. This overlapping can cause confusion and anxiety on the part of the employees. In one recorded case, the LPNs of the hospital were in direct charge of evaluating the aides and orderlies working for them; and in an organizing campaign, certain prounion LPNs threatened the aides or orderlies with bad ratings if they did not assist in getting the union in the hospital.

Supervisors in hospitals are often well educated in modern health care techniques and training methods; but they rarely receive any training in the human relations side of health care supervision, which is another problem in hospitals. As a result, many hospital supervisors are excellent at the technical aspects of their jobs but are too insensitive to their subordinate employees.

The other side of the same problem is that lower level supervisors in a hospital might empathize so closely with employees that the supervisor will actually assist the union organizing campaign, or even openly attend union meetings. Such conduct certainly justifies the termination of such supervisors.

Communications Audit

The day of the attitude survey is about over. Historically, attitude surveys produced only symptoms and opportunities for negativism. The communications audit, therefore, has been developed to discover interruptions in the flow of both informal and formal communication channels. It is possible through a communications audit, to see the communications network within the health care institution and to pinpoint basic problems, not external symptoms.

In some large hospitals, isolation and alienation become the rule rather than the exception. In the authors' experience, communication audits have revealed that workers often feel like a third hand, useful, but not necessary. The employee feels powerless as an object being controlled and manipulated by other persons in an impersonal work system. If such a worker feels that the system cannot be changed he/she becomes prime bait for unionization.

It is beyond the scope of this book to go into the specific techniques of the audit, but there are a number of excellent references available in the libraries, or one might consider using the services of an independent consultant specializing in such an area. Beyond the communications audit and consultants there are a number of ways by which you can now open channels of communication.

IMPROVING COMMUNICATIONS

Review Your Communications

Take a look at your communications to your employees. This includes your policies, your memos, your bulletin board messages, and so on. Do they read like a Department of Health, Education, and Welfare regulation? If so, it is no wonder that employees do not understand hospital policies. Do your communications reflect the "feel" of the organization or do they reflect stagnation? Do they inform or preach? Are they meaningful or meaningless? Do they consider the human interest or take the employee into account? Most importantly, do they encourage feedback?

Encouraging Feedback

A major problem in most health care organizations is the lack of employee feedback. It is interesting to note that in most of our advanced technological computer systems, over sixty-five percent of the system functions to check its own reliabilities. Sadly in management, we often tell the employee as little as possible and as firmly as possible. If we want feedback, and you should, you must:

1. Listen to all the employee is saying. Do not interrupt to explain or justify your action. If you ask for employee feedback, the burden is on you to listen and try to understand.

2. Request more information from employees. When you do have an opportunity to get more information or feedback from an employee, you can help the process by simply saying, "That is really helpful, can you tell me more?" Or, "Is there anything else I should know?"

3. Make employee feedback a way of life. If the feedback is negative, accept it as being an honest reaction of the individual employee providing it. Express and acknowledge your appreciation for the employee discussing it with you. Do not use it as an excuse to "jump down the employee's throat."

Broadcast—Don't Just Receive

All too often management is guilty of receiving all the communications upward and never reversing the flow by broadcasting. Employees are interested in what management has to say, particularly its reaction to current problems and issues facing employees or the hospital. Naturally those at the top should be informed as to what is going on, but they should never forget to furnish employees with their side of the "two way street" of communications.

Face to Face Communication

It is a fact that for maximum understanding, face to face communication is the most effective. Too often supervisors become "desk jockeys" and sit behind their two-penned desks, nursing stations, or executive office doors and issue directives, never getting to the floors where the action is.

In all communications, supervisors should use as many channels as they possibly can. If the employee can hear it, see it, touch it, taste it, or even smell it, the communication is going to be more effective. When messages can stimulate multiple senses, the receiver has a variety of reinforcing signals that help greatly to reduce message interference. For example, an employee hearing a message from his/her boss and seeing it in writing has twice the opportunity for confirmation of message content.

Reduce Status Awareness and Social Distance

One of the major barriers to communication in health care is the perceived necessity to maintain social distance and status by imposing such barriers as artificial titles. Status differences are always going to be with you, but if you are to have effective communications and substantially reduce the chances for unionization you need to try to reduce status symbols. How many times have you heard, "why, if I let my people call me by my first name they wouldn't have any respect for me." If you have a prestigious title this tends to be even more ominous. The end result is that the supervisor is seen as a "title" not a person, and who wants to go to a title with a problem?

We can learn from union organizers by the way they work. They consistently approach the employee on an informal basis, always using their first name, and often with the result that they get more production out of them in a short campaign than a supervisor can get out of the same individual in a year. Respect is not conferred with a title; it must be earned.

Get to Know Your Employees

Getting to know your employees is not only a primary necessity for effective communications but for good management as well. In the authors' experience it has been the rare individual that knows his/her employees on a first name basis. Many say they do but it reality don't. You might want to give yourself the following test:

1. What are the first names of all employees that work for you?
2. What is the name of each employee's spouse?
3. How many children does each have, and what grades are they in?
4. What major illnesses have occurred in the employee's family recently?
5. What hobbies does each of your employees have?
6. What educational or vocational courses has each of them taken?
7. Where does each of the employees live? (Not by street address or number, but in what section of town.)
8. How long does it take for each to get to work, and how does each get to work?

If you took the above quiz and did not know the answers to at least 5 or 6 questions about each employee under your supervision then you are a prime target for a union because you don't really know your employees. Do not make the fatal error of falling back on the lame excuse of "well, I don't know names, but I can remember faces." Research has indicated this isn't the case. One of the authors recently conducted an experiment using fifty executives attending a "memory training" seminar. Photographs of employees who had worked for the managers, many working currently, were flashed on the screen together with faces of employees that worked elsewhere. Also, included were faces of people with whom the group had been in conference three weeks earlier. The conferees were asked to name the people shown on the projection

screen. If they were unable to name them then they were to identify faces that were familiar. The group failed miserably. The
average manager could only name those with whom he/she was
having current contact and only by the last name. In addition,
they often identified faces they had never seen as being a "face I
could never forget."

The point is to care enough to know your employees. If you
don't, the union will.

IMPROVING SUPERVISION

The employee in a health care facility is represented by his/her
immediate supervisor. In every case when a hospital goes union,
considerable blame can be placed at the feet of poor supervision.
For example, many of the barriers to effective communication can
be overcome only with the help of effective supervisory participation. There are four primary ways to improve supervision.

Develop a Good Selection Procedure

The selection of personnel for a health care organization is a
difficult process that involves the matching of the abilities, ap-
titudes, interests, and personalities of applicants against the
specifications of the job. Management should use every possible
tool to get the right person on the right job. Such tools include
development of current and accurate job specifications and job
descriptions. Management also needs data about the applicant
for the position, whether the applicant is coming from within or
outside of the hospital. Such data can be obtained from the application form, references (that have been validated), background
checks, credit reports, validated personality tests, and in-depth in-
terviews with the applicant.

It is important to match the right person with the right job. If
you put a good person in a mediocre job, you can count on
developing a mediocre person.

Provide Sound Supervisory Training

Unfortunately, too much time is devoted to skills training in
hospitals as opposed to supervisory human relations training.

When supervisory training is offered it is too often the same time-worn material. It will tell us in what block a person is or should be and what kind of carrot will motivate (actually manipulate) an employee to pull a cart. Seldom is a health care periodical or piece of management literature be published without reference to the two-factor theory, the one that says basically, "money doesn't motivate." Yet such research has been proven to be wrong and full of methodological error time and time again—which just goes to show that things are often said because they can be said well, not because they are based on fact.

Good management training teaches a manager how to manage in the present situation as well as in the future. Discussion of the X and Y theory, the managerial grid (which is the same thing) is a good training aid, but it will seldom develop good supervisory personnel.

On the other hand, communication skills and interpersonal skills training can offer supervisory management the opportunity to develop. It is interesting to note that Transactional Analysis (TA), which is thought to be new but is really as old as Aristotle, has been of immense use in management development. TA is a practical and useful system of understanding interpersonal relationships. In reality it is simplified psychology and, as clinicians are finding out, more effective than classifcal psychology. It is easy to learn and provides a positive communication tool that is immediately usable. It increases a supervisor's on the job effectiveness by providing better insights into personalities and transactions that occur between people. Most important, it is a non-threatening approach to self evaluation and offers a method for not only analyzing people scripts but scripts of organizations as well.

Unfortunately, there are too few qualified people to teach TA in organizations. There are many who try after reading books such as, *I'm OK—You're OK, Born to Win, Games People Play,* etc. These popular books all give an excellent, though superficial, insight into TA but fail to provide the requirements for teaching in a management development situation. The health care manager should watch for the "instant consultant" or the "mini-shrink," who claims to be a management consultant in everything. This, of course, would apply to any consultant who would be considered to be hired to work in your organization. It is sometimes better to pay a little more and get quality than to skimp and get a union.

Management training is extremely vital. If in-house capability is not present, and often it is not due to the prohibitive cost, then consider outside sources such as local universities, qualified consultants, or attend top-notch seminars that are periodically offered by quality organizations such as the American Management Association, Aspen Systems Corporation, etc. Remember that good management is a skill that must be developed. Few people are born with the natural ability necessary to supervise effectively.

Develop Good Supervisory Evaluation

The supervisor who does not listen, does not talk, does not develop his/her people, and does not care will stay that way unless corrected in a formal evaluation. Such a supervisor is a liability to any organization. Surprisingly there are many hospitals that still have no form of supervisory evaluation, or if they do, it is more perfunctory than practical in nature. A supervisor should receive a rating on a minimum of every six months, but the standard is more likely once a year or not at all.

Maintain High Supervisory Involvement

Getting supervisors into decision-making is essential. To do this involves keeping the supervisors (at all levels of management) informed as to the status of the current operations, providing sources of two-way communications, and periodically getting them involved in the decision-making and goal-setting processes.

The benefits are several. A manager who is part of the decision-making process has more invested in reaching that decision, as does a manager who takes part in the setting of a goal. He has more invested in the achievement of that goal. By the same token, a manager who is involved in creativity has more invested in the outcome of what is created.

DEVELOP A GOOD GRIEVANCE PROCEDURE

Employees who feel helpless to change their working situation are fertile territory for unionization. They feel they are the victims of the system, and management is the persecutor. A union organizer then convinces them that the union can be the liberator by promising the installation of a grievance procedure whereby employees can be guaranteed a fair deal in a management/labor conflict. Every health care organization will benefit if it develops and uses a grievance procedure before any union activity commences. The authors have noted that in many successful unionization campaigns, the hospital did not have or did not use such procedures.

To be effective a grievance procedure should include:

1. A simple written account of the grievance procedure.

2. Varying steps of appeal (usually three is sufficient) through which the employee can seek regress for his/her perceived unfair treatment.

3. Alternate routes of appeal which can be taken by an employee should he/she feel the need to bypass an immediate supervisor. Ordinarily the personnel department is the alternate route. Figure 1 presents an example of a grievance system that might exist in a hospital for the nursing department.

4. A time limit must be set for each step, so management is prohibited from delaying the processing of a complaint. This requires the grievance system to have total support of all management, to avoid the possibility of it becoming just a formality for approving management actions. The grievance (large or small) must be acted on in all cases. This is necessary for the system to build integrity.

5. An appeal mechanism for both management and employees. If an employee is turned down on the initial appeal or if management feels that the decision was truly unfair, each should have the right to continue on to the next appeal.

6. A final review board for arbitration, containing employees as well as management personnel. True representation must

be provided. If employee representation is not provided, then employees usually view the whole grievance process as a mere rubber stamp for the supervisor.

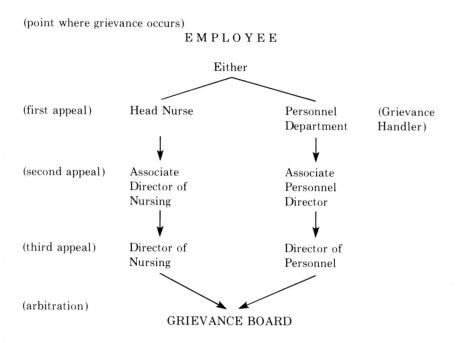

(point where grievance occurs)

EMPLOYEE

Either

(first appeal)   Head Nurse   Personnel   (Grievance
                            Department   Handler)

(second appeal) Associate   Associate
                Director of   Personnel
                Nursing   Director

(third appeal)   Director of   Director of
                Nursing   Personnel

(arbitration)

GRIEVANCE BOARD

NURSING DEPARTMENT GRIEVANCE PROCEDURE

In small organizations a grievance committee or a board of neutral individuals (individuals without vested interest in the outcome) could substitute for a formal grievance procedure. Sometimes an "open door" policy can be used effectively, whereby any employee is free to talk to any level of supervision and express grievances. Though the "open door" policy sounds great and is widely advertised to employees by many managers, especially around union election time, it seldom works. Managers too often feel "bound" to support their supervisors, and they should to a certain extent. Consequently, the final decision process for resolving grievances is best left in the hands of those further removed from the questioned action, and those without vested interests.

DEVELOP GOOD EMPLOYEE EVALUATION AND SALARY ADMINISTRATION POLICIES

Often in a union election campaign, the union will raise complaints about the hospital's pay and promotion policies. Employee evaluation is frequently never done or poorly done. The problem here, of course, is that many hospitals have never faced the responsibility for employee evaluation.

Much of the time an employee is rated on the basis of personality traits, which have little to do with job performance. To compound this problem, job performance is seldom related to pay, so the basic problem becomes evident. The employee is supposed to get paid for the work he/she performs; there should be a connection between pay and work. If there isn't, a natural discrepancy and bad morale most likely will result. The following is a summary of steps of a pay evaluation procedure that the authors have used with great success in various organizations.

1. With input from the employee, develop performance requirements. Both the employee and supervisor should determine how well the employee is expected to do his/her duties.
2. When finalized, discuss the performance requirements with the employee and adjust them periodically, upon mutual agreement, as needed.
3. Observe and discuss current employee performance.
4. The employee's performance should be evaluated against his/her performance requirements.
5. The results of the evaluation must always be discussed with the employee.
6. Action should be taken as a result of the evaluation. Such action could be corrective or advisory in nature, or a raise of pay if justified.

Additional elements that serve to make a good pay-evaluation program include a period of evaluation not less that once a year, with twice or three times being even better. Expectations should be known by both parties (supervisor and employee) and agreed upon in advance of the evaluation. Ordinarily it is good to develop these in writing for the benefit of the employee, as well as the supervisor, and to get consenting signatures.

An appeal process should be available to any employee who is dissatisfied with his evaluation. Ordinarily this can be the grievance procedure system. It is a good idea to get the evaluation commented on or reviewed by the next level of supervision. Any discrepancy between levels of supervision should be reconciled, which is best done by the remaining levels of management. Finally, there should be a written performance review, which should contain positive as well as any negative areas. When negative evaluative criteria are present, corrective action should be given. Such corrective action is best developed by the immediate supervisor and the employee together.

The performance evaluation, when done correctly, can be a powerful tool for employee development. It can also become one the of the mainstays for preventive unionism.

DEVELOP FAIR JOB PROMOTION AND JOB TRANSFER POLICIES

Most of the major corporations in the United States long ago recognized the importance of fair job promotion and job transfer policies. They recognized that it is important for an employee not only to know his/her present status within the organization but also the opportunities available within the organization. One method to accomplish this is through job posting.

Job posting is a system whereby all available jobs are posted on a bulletin board. Employees are given this opportunity so they can indicate that they might have an interest in a particular job. Personnel screens the applicants and refers those who are qualified. Each applicant is then notified regarding his/her application for the job and the final action that was taken.

Such a procedure provides the worker with the opportunity of applying for any new position with the same privileges as an "outsider." As often happens, we look outside our organizations for replacements without considering those inside. It is too easy to say, "we do not have anyone qualified." It is more honest to admit that we may be too lazy to even look.

Frequently, the causes of unionism include the lack of clarity and enforcement of management policies relating to promotion and job transfer. Sometimes these policies seem "hit and miss." This gives the employee a feeling of hopelessness, which is increased if he/she sees better jobs going to "newcomers" who are not necessarily the best qualified. It is important for managers to realize that often good employees are not recommended for promotion because their first line supervisor does not want to lose good people. Management must wage a campaign to win the loyalty of its employees and to turn its "lip service" actions into actual practice.

CONSIDER A RESTRUCTURING OF THE ORGANIZATION

Without a doubt, the structure of an organization influences the relationships within that organization. As health care facilities grow in size, they tend to become impersonal, leaving the employee feeling like a pawn in a huge game of chess. He/she feels far removed from the decision-making process and from those controlling his/her welfare. Oddly enough the same feeling is engendered in managers. With both management and non-management feeling isolated it is no small wonder that communication problems exist and that unionization attempts begin. There are a number of ways management can reduce these dilemmas. The organizational structure of the health care facility might need to be restructured to reduce possible built-in conflicts.

Try Job Enrichment/Enlargement

Job enrichment or enlargement procedures are high-sounding names, which might make a hospital supervisor feel the expert services of the most qualified management consultant or industrial engineer available are required. Such is not the case. Some methods of job enlargement/enrichment are within the realm of every supervisor:

1. Removing some of the management controls over people without removing accountability. By doing this, personal achievement is stimulated within the employees.

2. Providing additional authority, thus giving an employee more opportunity to make decisions. This means increasing job freedom within the job itself. The motivators of responsibility, achievement, and recognition are powerfully stimulated when job freedom is increased.

3. Increasing employees' accountability for their own work.

4. Giving employees a whole natural unit of work to do when possible. Make them responsible for doing it. In many ways we have become too mass-production-minded. The Vega automobile plant realized that in 1972 when their workers went on strike to rebel against mind-confining jobs, e.g., attaching 8,000 bolts to a fender per day. The more complete a job a worker can do, the more achievement-oriented that worker will tend to be.

5. Making informational or periodical reports and the like available to the employee. In this way the employee is made to feel "in on things."

6. Introducing new and more difficult tasks to employees from time to time. These should be tasks that have not been previously handled by the employee, stimulating growth and learning.

7. Assigning specific or specialized tasks to employees from time to time to help them become experts in an area. This not only stimulates growth and learning but motivates the employee for advancement as well.

Job enrichment/enlargement is an excellent way to build up worker morale by increasing the number of intrinsic rewards gained from work activity. Such rewards gained from the work itself are far more satisfying than a supervisor's "pat on the head."

Reduce the Numbers of Levels of Supervision

Considerable research has proven that professional organizations function better when the management hierarchy is limited.

There is no magic number of people who can or should report to a supervisor. You often hear the number "ten," but that is just a myth. The number depends largely on the jobs being done by the employees, the communication required between supervision and employees, and the strengths of the supervisors.

Obviously, if there are ten employees all doing totally separate jobs and each requiring approval of the supervisor, even that number could be too many. On the other hand, if twenty people are doing similar jobs and a minimum amount of actual supervision of activities is required, then the number of employees within the span of management can be increased.

SUMMARY

Chapter 7 began with a listing of promises commonly made by unions during an election campaign. The thesis being, if unions are promising better working conditions, increased benefits, and wages and employees feel that they can only get these needs fulfilled by voting union, why doesn't management fulfill the promises first?

Unions realize that if there are no problems in communications and if management follows sound practices, they do not have a very good chance of organizing. As you have learned in the preceding chapters, the organizers spend a considerable amount of their time seeking out the problems in health care organizations to exploit management's weaknesses or management's failures. If unions promise employees that they have the remedy for management's failures, then it is only logical to assume that management can implement that remedy and do it first.

Specifically, this chapter has recommended that the health care facility: (a) consider a communications audit to determine its current problems in communications; (2) improve communications through review and feedback, maintaining open communication by both broadcasting and receiving, using multimedia communication, and reducing status awareness and social distance; (3) get to really know your employees as individuals; (4) improve supervision through good selection, training, evaluation, and involvement; (5) develop fair grievance procedures; (6) develop good employee evaluation and salary administration policies, as well as good job promotion and transfer policies; and (7) consider restructuring the organization through job enlargement and reduction of the management hierarchy.

In summary, though these suggested remedies might appear to be defensive they should represent those things we would want to do, not because we fear any union, but because we are interested in the employee and the enhancement of health care that will benefit the patient as a result of the mature development of all the organization's supervisors and employees.

NOTE

1. C.S. Golden and H. J. Ruttenberg, *The Dynamics of Industrial Democracy* 3 (2nd. ed. 1942).

Glossary of Labor Terms

Administrative Law Judge — Person who conducts the hearing on unfair labor practice complaints. Independent of both the National Labor Relations Board and the Office of the General Counsel.

Agency's Shop — A contract clause requiring nonmembers of a union to pay a sum equal to union dues to the union or a designated party.

Arbitration — A method by which the employer and the union agree to submit their disputes to a third party for binding resolution.

Authorization Card — A card signed by an employee designating the union as exclusive bargaining agent of the employee.

Back Pay — Lost wages required to be paid to employees discharged illegally under the National Labor Relations Act.

Boycott — A refusal to buy the products of a business as a means of exercising economic pressure in a labor dispute.

Business Agent — Paid representative of an international union or a local union who handles negotiations with employers, organizing new members, and other union business matters.

Captive Audience Speech — Speech delivered by an employer on its premises regarding the union, especially if all employees are required to attend.

Card Check — Verifying the written authorization cards signed by employees against the employer's signature records to determine whether the union truly represents a majority of the employees.

Cease and Desist Order — Order issued by the National Labor Relations Board requiring an employer or union to abstain from commission of an unfair labor practice. Such orders can only be enforced through the United States Court of Appeals.

Certification. — The official designation by the National Labor Relations Board of a labor union as the exclusive bargaining representation of employees in a certain unit.

Charge — Formal allegations filed under oath against an employer or a union alleging violations of the National Labor Relations Act.

Check-Off — Contract clause by which an employer periodically deducts from the pay of the employee the amount of union dues and remits the proceeds to the union.

Closed Shop — An arrangement between an employer and union under which only members of the union can be hired.

Collective Bargaining — Negotiations between a union and employer for a written labor contract covering the terms and working conditions of employees.

Concerted Activities — Activities undertaken jointly by two or more employees for the purposes of union organization, collective bargaining, mutual presentation of grievances, or other mutual job actions.

Conciliation — A nonbinding effort by a third party toward the accommodation of two opposing viewpoints to effect a voluntary settlement of a labor dispute.

Consent Election — When the employer and the union agree to waive hearing and agree to proceed by informal election machinery. There are two types of informal adjustments: (1) the agreement for consent election and (2) the stipulation for certification upon consent election. The latter is usually preferred.

Constructive Discharge — Where an employer marks an employee for discharge and creates such unfavorable treatment to the employee that he is forced to "voluntarily" resign from his employment.

Consumer Picketing — Picketing in support of a strike action at a retail level in which the pickets ask that customers not patronize the store or buy a particular product sold by the store.

Cooling-Off-Period — A ten-day notice period provided by law, required before a union can strike a hospital, in which time it is hoped a settlement can be reached.

Craft Union — A bargaining union usually consisting of employees in the construction industry such as carpenters, boilermakers, steel workers, and others.

Decertification Petition — Filed by a group of employees before the National Labor Relations Board to determine whether the employees wish to withdraw bargaining authority from the existing union by a NLRB-conducted vote of such employees..

Discharge — The permanent termination of an employee by an employer.

Discrimination — The National Labor Relations Act forbids all forms of discrimination in regard to hiring or tenure of employment as a means of encouraging or discouraging membership in any labor organization.

Discriminatory Discharge — A discharge in violation of Section 8(a)(3) of the act because it is based, in part, upon the union activity of such employee.

Domination — Illegal interference or control by an employer of the affairs of a labor organization.

Economic Strike — A strike caused by the failure of an employer to agree to a union's demand for wages, fringe benefits, or other terms and conditions of employment, rather than a strike provoked by an unfair labor practice of an employer.

Emergency Dispute — A strike or labor dispute which would imperil the national health and safety. In this case special procedures are provided under the National Labor Relations Act.

Employee Association — A grouping of employees that might or might not qualify as a labor union under the NLRA.

Employee Election — Secret balloting conducted under the supervision of the National Labor Relations Board for employees to determine the choice of a bargaining agent or the rejection of the one previously recognized.

Employee Representation Plan — Various systems under which the employees select part of the representatives to a joint body with hospital management, the purpose being either to discuss grievances or various company policies and benefits.

Employer Association — A joint grouping of employers in related enterprises, usually acting together as a single bargaining unit with one or more labor unions.

Employer Unit — A bargaining unit consisting of all or certain groupings of employees working for a single employer, even though in numerous locations.

Employment Contract — A written agreement entered into between an employee and employer covering the terms and conditions of such employment.

Equal Employment Opportunity Act — A federal law giving the Equal Employment Opportunity Commission authority to bring suits in federal district courts against employers or unions where it finds reasonable cause to believe that there has been discrimination based on race, color, religion, sex, or national origin.

Escalator Clause — A clause in a collective bargaining contract requiring wage or salary adjustments at timed intervals based on some ratio to changes in the Consumer Price Index, or some other inflationary indicator.

Escape Clause — A period, normally a few days, during which an employee can resign from a union without being bound to continue dues, whether under check-off or membership-maintenance agreements.

Espionage — An illegal employer practice of spying on employees to discover memberships in or activities on behalf of a labor union.

Fair Employment Practice — A term applied in approval of conduct that does not contravene any of the prohibitions against discrimination in employment because of race, color, religion, sex, or national origin.

Featherbedding — A contractual requirement that employees be hired in excessive numbers for services that are not needed.

Fink — One who continues to work in a struck hospital or becomes employed in a hospital during a strike.

Free Rider — A term usually applied by a union to nonmembers within the bargaining unit who do not pay union dues and are still entitled to the benefits of a collective bargaining contract.

Free Speech — The specific provision of the National Labor Relations Act guaranteeing the right of employers to express views hostile to unionization.

Fringe Benefits — A term usually applied to all benefits in addition to the direct wages provided employees. It includes such items as vacations, holidays, sick pay, insurance benefits, pension benefits, and other similar benefits.

Furlough — A layoff period from work.

General Counsel's Office — An office independent from the National Labor Relations Board whose chief duty is to issue and prosecute complaints and unfair labor practice cases, which are presented to the National Labor Relations Board for decision.

Good Faith Bargaining — The bargaining obligation imposed under the National Labor Relations Act on both the employer and the union to meet at reasonable times and to confer in good faith with respect to wages, hours, and other terms and conditions of employment.

Grievance — A complaint or allegation by an employee, union, or employer that a collective bargaining contract provision has been violated.

Grievance Committee — A committee selected by the employees or designated by a union to meet with hospital management to discuss grievances.

Independent Union — Usually refers to a local labor union, not affiliated with a nationally organized union or a national federation of unions.

Informational Picketing — Picketing for the purpose of advising the public that the picketed employer does not have a union contract or is selling goods produced by a struck or nonunion employer.

Initiation Fee — Fees required by labor unions as a condition of becoming members in such labor organizations.

International Union — A nationally organized labor union, having locals in various parts of the United States, sometimes also having locals in Canada or Mexico.

Intimidation — Actual, implied, or veiled threats to induce employees to refrain from joining or to join a labor union. Intimidation is illegal.

Judicial Review — Proceedings before the United States Court of Appeals for the enforcement or setting aside of orders issued by the National Labor Relations Board.

Jurisdiction — Statutory and self-imposed jurisdictional standards of the National Labor Relations Board on the size and involvement of an employer in interstate commerce.

Jurisdictional Dispute — The disagreement between two unions over whose members shall be employed on a specific type of work or over the right to organize a given class or group of employees.

Jurisdictional Strike — A strike called by one union to compel an employer to assign work to one class or craft of employees rather than to another group.

Labor Contract — A written and binding legal contract entered into between an employer and a labor organization covering employees' wages, hours, and other terms and conditions of employment.

Labor Dispute — Under the terms of the Norris-LaGuardia Act, the statute was narrowly drawn as a limitation on the jurisdiction of the federal courts to issue injunctions in certain defined labor disputes.

Labor/Management Relations Act of 1947 — A major amendment to the labor law defining labor union unfair labor practices.

Labor/Management Reporting and Disclosure Act of 1959 — A major amendment to the labor law establishing a Code of Conduct for labor unions, union officers, employers, and labor relations consultants. Also, certain reporting procedures were made mandatory. Also known as the Landrum-Griffin Act.

Labor Relations Board — The same as the National Labor Relations Board.

Labor Union — An organization representing employees for the purposes of dealing with the employer concerning grievances, labor disputes, wages, rates of pay, hours of employment, or conditions of work.

Layoff — Removing an employee temporarily from the payroll, usually during a period of slack work with the intention of rehiring when needed.

Local — A group of organized employees holding a charter from a national or international labor organization. A local is usually confined to union members in one small locality, or of one employer.

Lockout — Where an employer voluntarily closes his business down as a form of economic pressure upon his employees to force acceptance of his contract terms or to prevent whipsawing by the union.

Maintenance of Membership — A union security agreement under which employees who are members of a union on a specified date, or thereafter become members, are required to remain members during the term of the contract as a condition of employment.

Majority Rule — A simple majority of the voters in representation elections determines whether the union will be the exclusive bargaining representative or not, as distinguished from a majority of those eligible to vote in the voting unit.

Management's Rights Clause — A contract clause that expressly reserves to management certain rights and benefits and so specifies that the exercise of these rights and benefits shall not be subject to the grievance procedure or arbitration.

Mandatory Injunction — Injunctions that the General Counsel's Office of the National Labor Relations Board is required to seek in certain cases of alleged unfair labor practices involving secondary boycotts, secondary recognition strikes, recognitional or organizational picketing, or strikes to force an employer to violate a National Labor Relations Board certification.

Mediation — Not binding on either party to a dispute, but an offer of the good offices of a third person who makes new proposals for the settlement of a dispute.

Mediation Service — Same as the Federal Mediation and Conciliation Service, which is a functional part of the settlement of disputes under the labor law.

Moonlighting — The practice of holding down two or more jobs at once.

Multiemployer Bargaining Unit — Where two or more employers join together in one single bargaining unit to deal with one or more labor unions.

National Labor Relations Act — Originally known as the Wagner Act and passed in 1935, amended by the Labor/Management Relations Act of 1947, also amended by the Landrum-Griffin Act in 1959, and amended in 1974.

Negotiating Committee — A committee selected by a union or an employer to negotiate on its behalf a collective bargaining contract.

Occupational Safety and Health Act — A federal law passed in 1970 giving the federal government authority to prescribe and enforce safety and health standards in most industries.

Open Shop — Where employees work and are free to join or not join any union.

Organizational Picketing — Picketing of an employer by a labor organization in an attempt to force employees to join the union.

Picketing — Signs usually carried by members of the union at an employer's site advertising the existence of a labor dispute and the union's version of it.

Professional Employee — Technical definition is provided in Section 2(12) of the National Labor Relations Act. This class of employee cannot be included in a unit containing nonprofessional employees, unless the professional employees so elect.

Professional Union — A labor union attempting to organize a specialty group of highly trained employees, such as registered nurses. It receives the same treatment under the National Labor Relations Act as any other labor union.

Publicity Picketing — Another term for picketing aimed at publicizing a particular aspect of a labor dispute.

Recognition — An employer acknowledging the labor union as the exclusive bargaining representative of its employees.

Recognitional Picketing — Picketing by a labor organization for the object of inducing or compelling the employer to recognize the union as the bargaining agent for all employees.

Regional Director — Local official of the National Labor Relations Board who serves in a specified regional area of the United States.

Reinstatement — The return to employment of persons unlawfully discharged under the National Labor Relations Act.

Representation Election — A National Labor Relations Board-conducted secret ballot election among the employees to determine whether they want to be represented by a labor organization.

Right to Work — A term used to describe state laws that ban certain union security agreements.

Sabotage — Malicious damage done to an employer's equipment or property during a labor dispute.

Scab — An employee who crosses the picket line to return to work while other employees are out on strike.

Secondary Boycott — The refusal to deal with or buy goods from an employer who is a customer or supplier of another employer with whom the boycotters have a primary dispute. It is a form of indirect pressure brought to bear on the primary employer.

Self-Organization — A group of employees who join together for the purpose of self-protective activity.

Seniority — The total length of service an employee has with a business and the certain preferences afforded such employee because of his length of service.

Shop Steward — An individual assigned by the union to present the grievances of his fellow employees to the employer.

Showing of Interest — The National Labor Relations Board requires that a union seeking a representation election make a showing of interest of at least thirty percent of the employees in the bargaining unit. Such showing of interest is usually provided by employee-signed union authorization cards.

Sit-Down Strike — Temporary stoppage of work when the striking employees remain in occupancy of the employer's premises.

Slowdown — A concerted slackening of the pace in work performance as a means of enforcing demands made by the employees.

Statute of Limitations — Unfair labor practice charges will not be received by the National Labor Relations Board if they are based on events that occurred more than six months ago.

Strike — A concerted effort by employees to cease all work as a form of economic pressure to enforce acceptance of their contract demands.

Strike Breaker — One who comes to work or begins employment during a strike situation.

Strike Vote — Balloting by employees on the decision to call a strike.

Subcontracting — Placing part of the hospital's work function with an outside employer.

Superseniority — A contract clause providing seniority in excess of what length of service would justify as a protection against a reduction of the work force. Union stewards are sometimes accorded superseniority.

Supervisor — Definition is provided in Section 2(11) of the National Labor Relations Act. Supervisors enjoy no protection of bargaining rights under the National Labor Relations Act.

Supplemental Unemployment Benefits — Employer-financed payments to laid off employees to supplement the state unemployment compensation benefits they receive.

Surveillance — Watching employees to detect their union organizing activites.

Taft-Hartley Act — A popular name for the National Labor Relations Act.

Unauthorized Strike — A strike called by employees contrary to the advice or without the consent of their labor union. Such strike can also be in direct violation of the labor contract.

Unfair Employment Practices — Any employment practice that results in discrimination in employment based on race, color, religion, sex, or national origin.

Unfair Labor Practice — Certain practices by both employers and unions that are declared to be illegal under the National Labor Relations Act.

Unfair Labor Practice Strike — A strike by employees that is either caused by or prolonged in whole or in part by the employer's unfair labor practice. In such a strike, the employer must reinstate the strikers in their jobs or equivalent jobs upon their unconditional application for that right.

Union Insignia — Buttons or other signs worn by employees to indicate that they are prounion.

Unit — An appropriate grouping of employees for purposes of collective bargaining.

Wagner Act — Popular name of the first federal labor law passed in 1935.

Walk-Out — Where the employees suddenly and without notice walk off their jobs.

Welfare and Pension Plan Disclosure Act — A federal law enacted in 1958, amended in 1962, that establishes reporting, disclosure, and regulatory requirements for almost all employee welfare, benefits, and pension plans.

Whipsawing — A labor union tactic where the union selects one weak employer in an area and calls a strike against that one employer to obtain a favorable contract. That contract is then presented to other employers in the area to accept.

Wildcat Strike — A strike by employees in violation of the labor contract and contrary to the advice or without the consent of their labor union.

Yellow Dog Contract — A written agreement whereby an employee undertakes not to join a labor union while working for his employer. This is unlawful under the National Labor Relations Act.

INDEX

About the Authors

Warren H. Chaney, Ph.D., is Assistant Professor of Health Care Administration and Management, the University of Houston at Clear Lake City in Houston, Texas. Additionally, he serves as a management consultant to major health care facilities as well as other business and industry organizations. Dr. Chaney has had broad experience in combating unionization attempts. His basic research into the causes and effects of labor organizations has received wide attention in such publications as the *Labor Law Journal*. His former positions include Director of Organizational Development, Western Company of North America; Director of Human Resources, World Trade Imports, Inc.; National Director of Sales Training, Frito-Lay, Inc.; Instructor, The Academy of Health Science; and an officer in the Medical Service Corps., United States Army.

Thomas R. Beech, J.D., has his law office in Houston, Texas and has represented numerous health care clients. He formerly served in the Honors Program, Office of the General Counsel, National Labor Relations Board, Washington, D.C. He has taught courses in Labor Law and Employee Rights at South Texas College of Law. Mr. Beech is a member of the American Society of Hospital Attorneys, American Bar Association, and numerous other professional associations.